Amazing Fireworks

Stunning Displays of Pyrotechnics

Curated by Pablo Rissen

ISBN-13: 978-1726278140
ISBN-10: 172627814X

Printed in the United States of America

First Edition

1 2 3 4 5 6 7 8 9 10

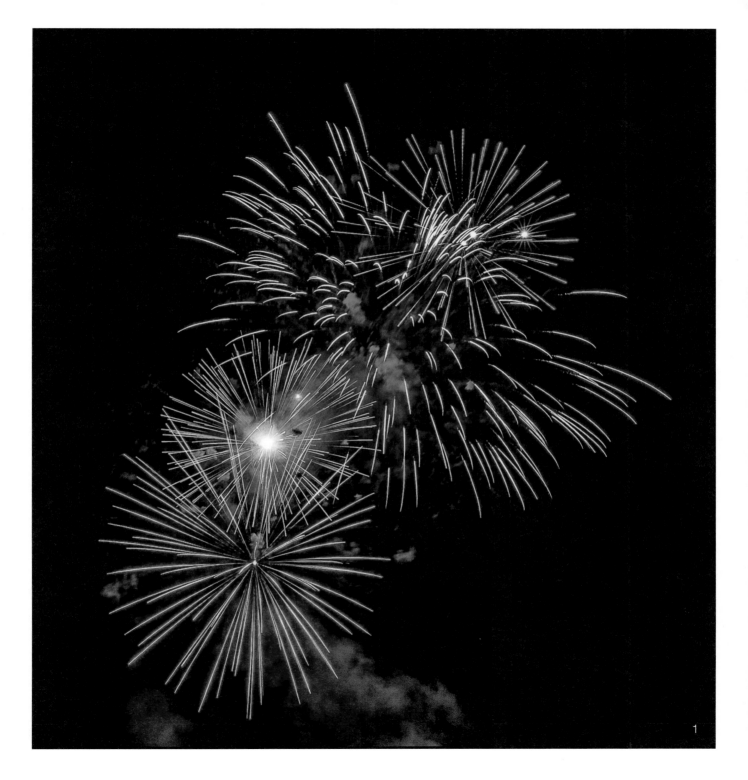

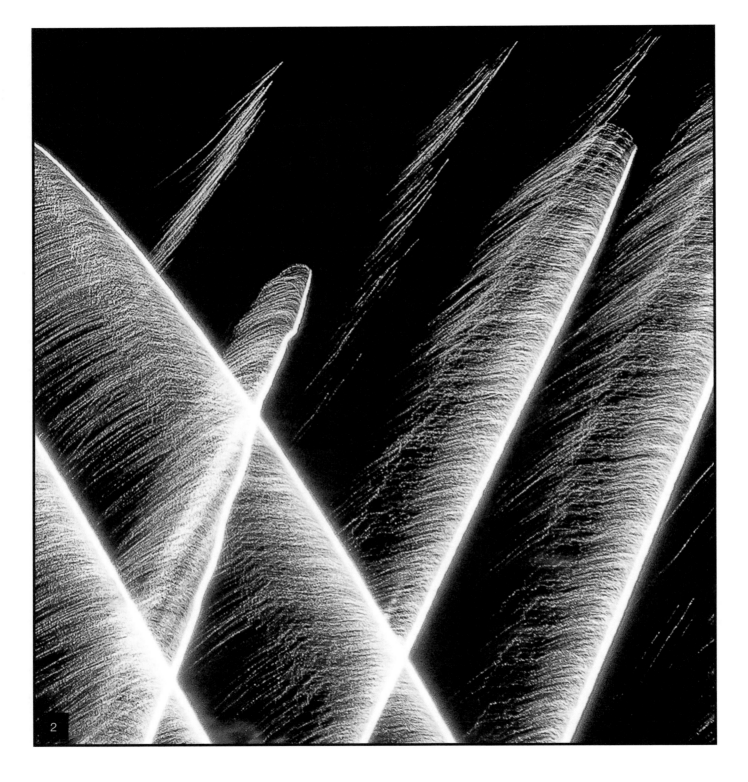

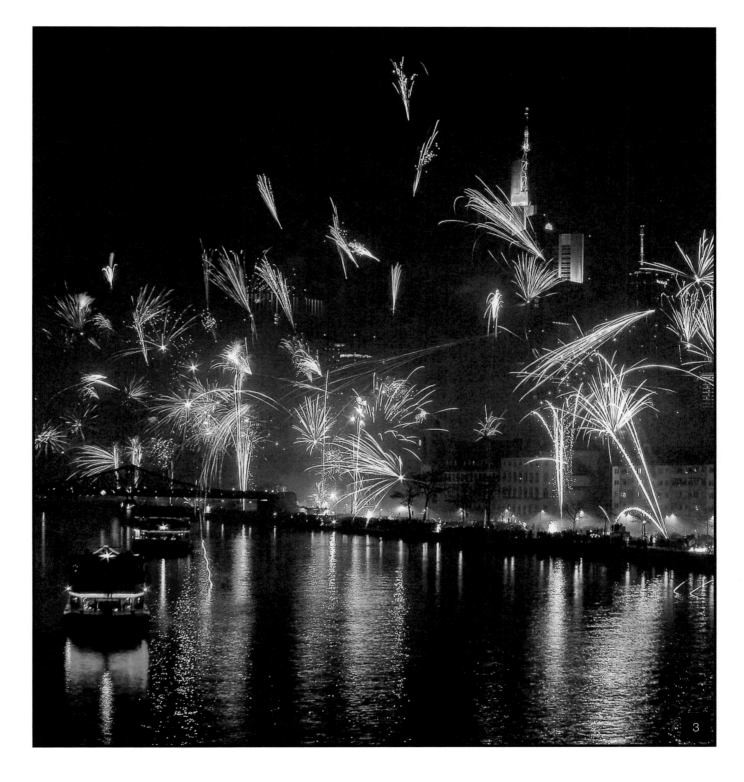
3

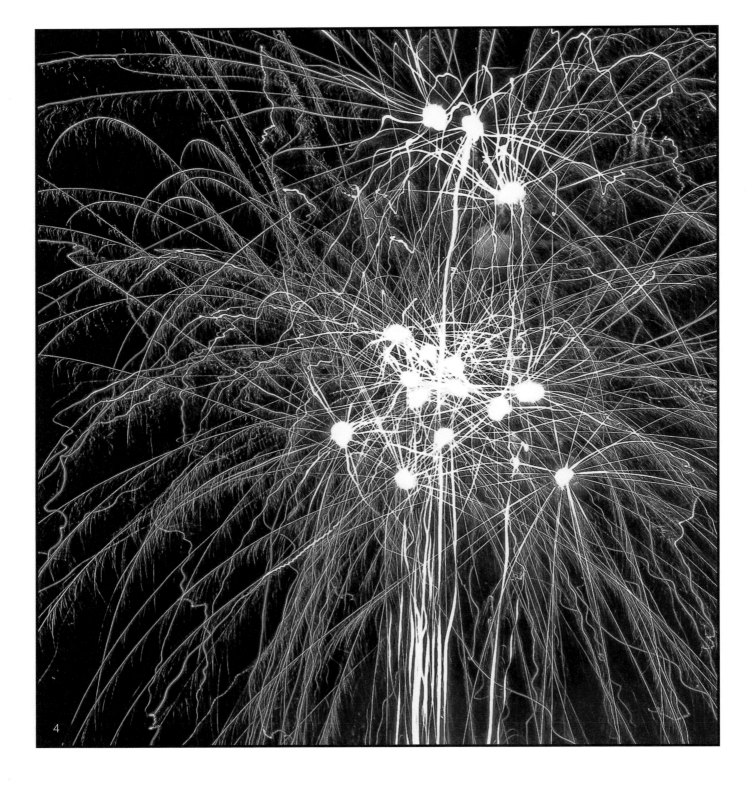

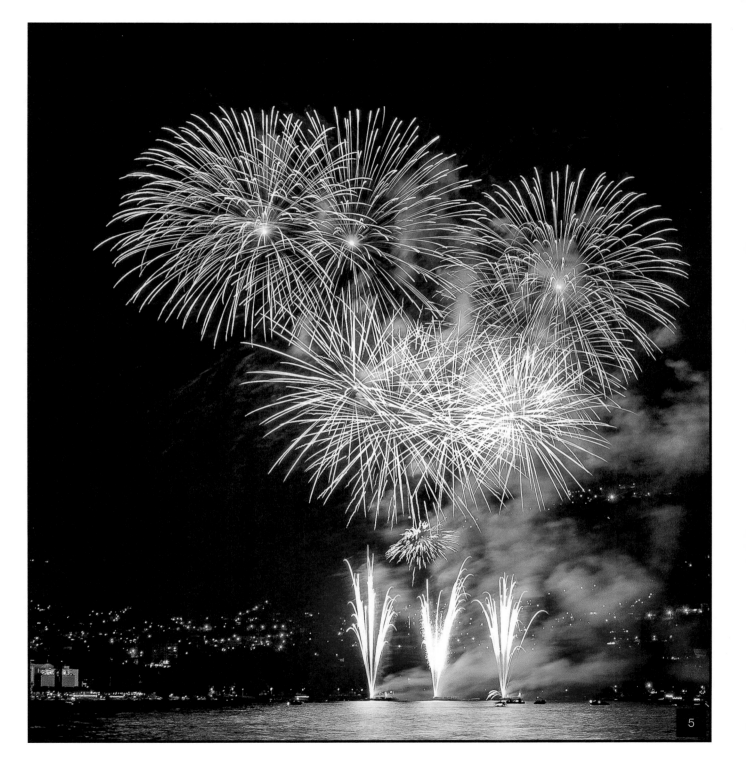

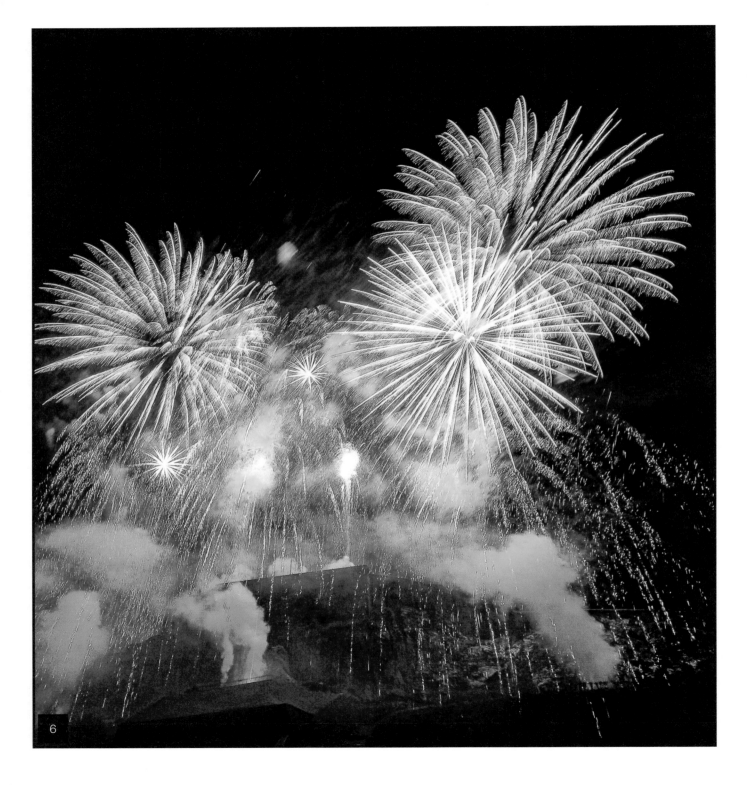

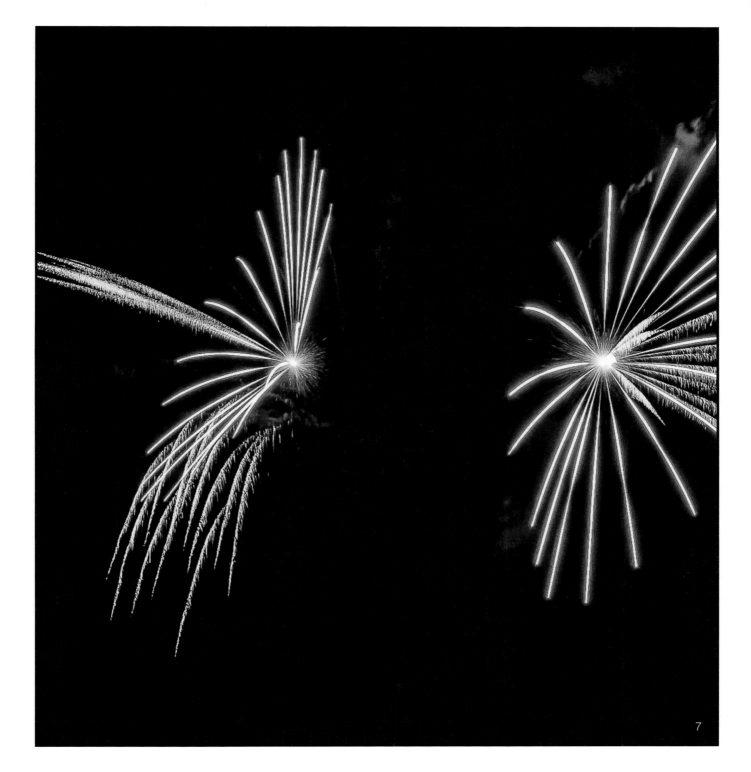

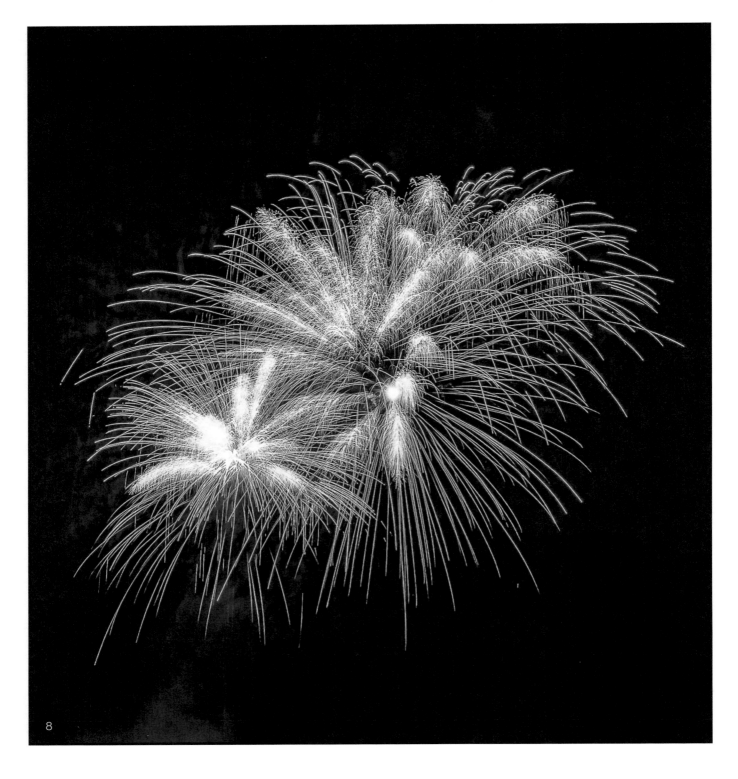

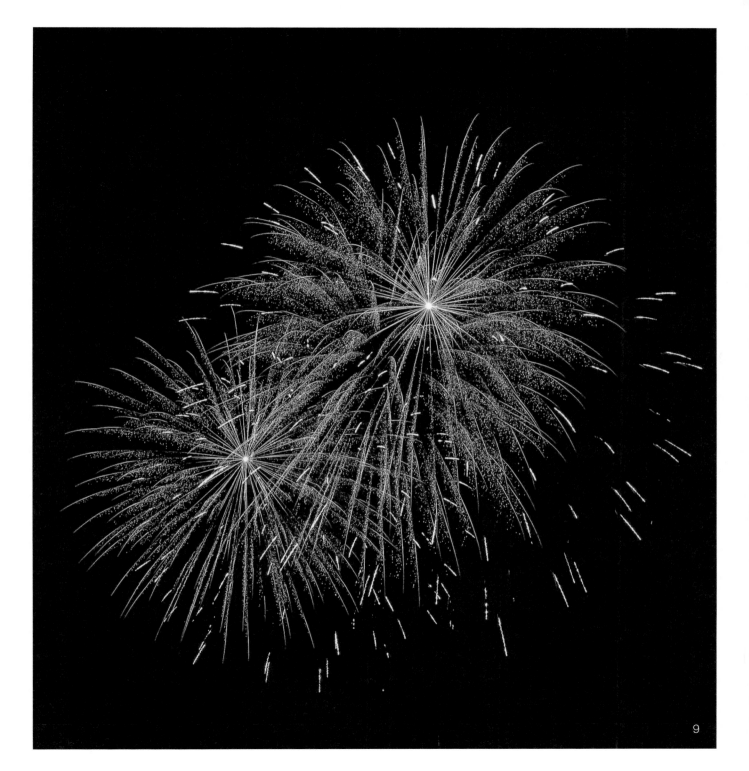

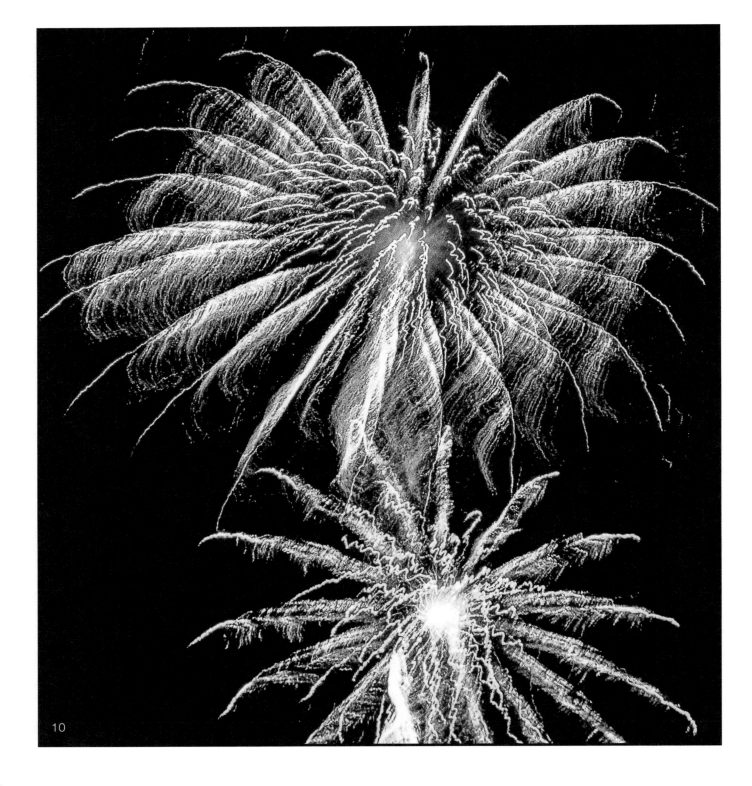

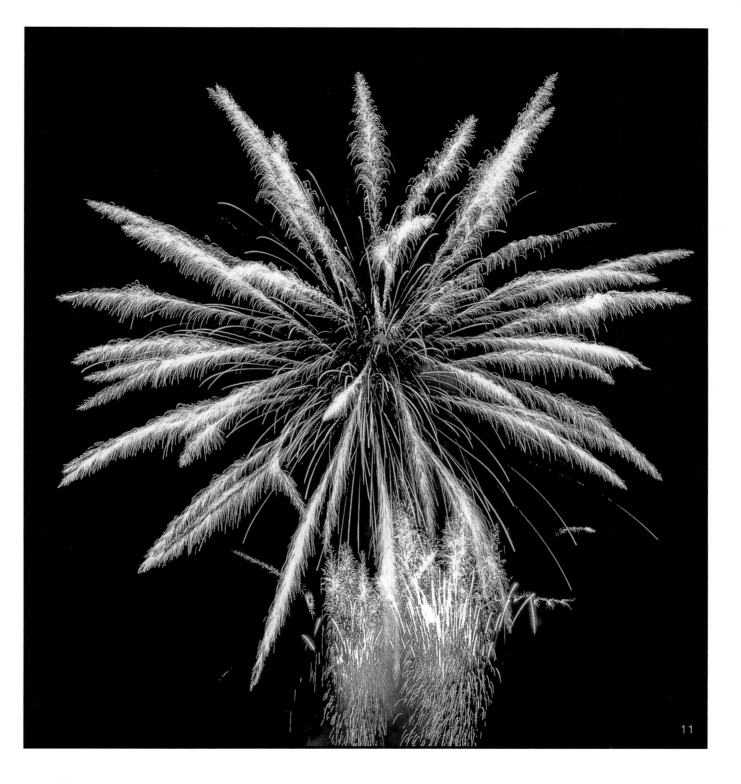

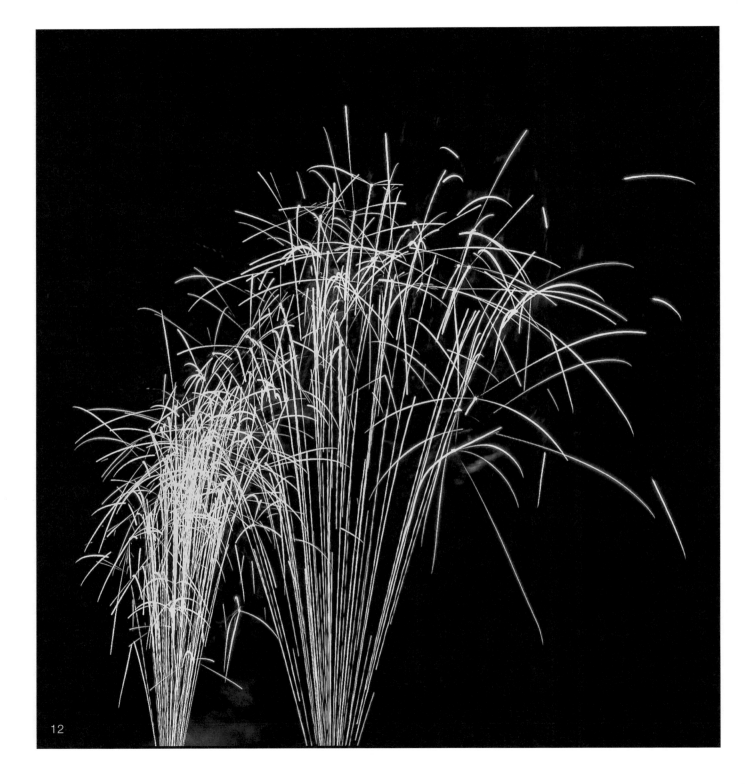

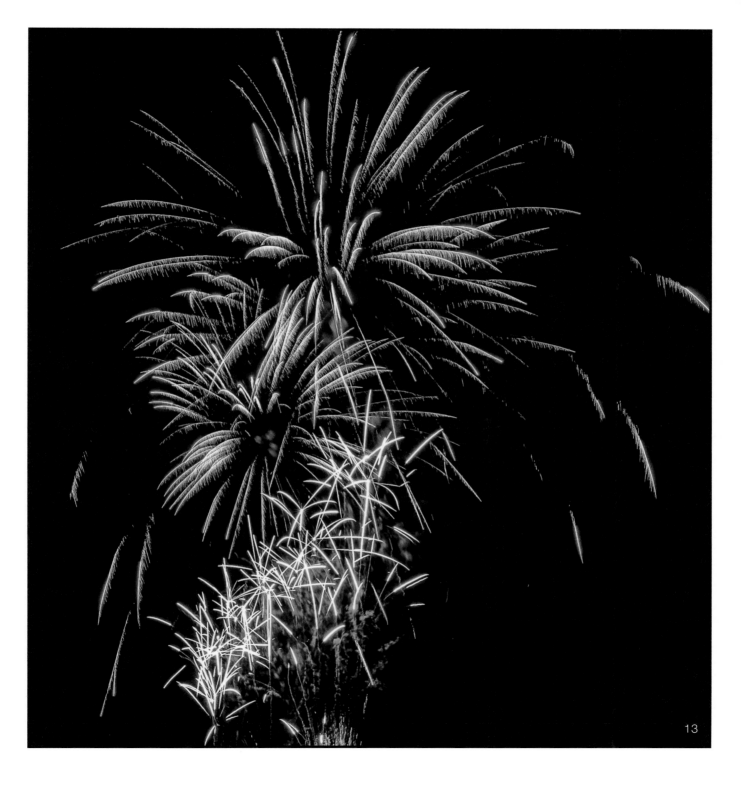

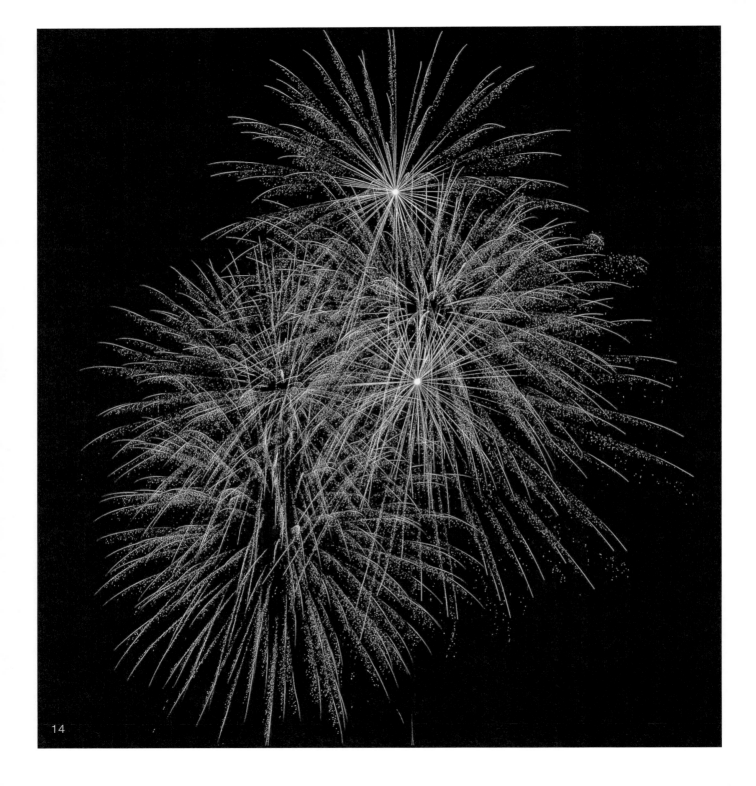

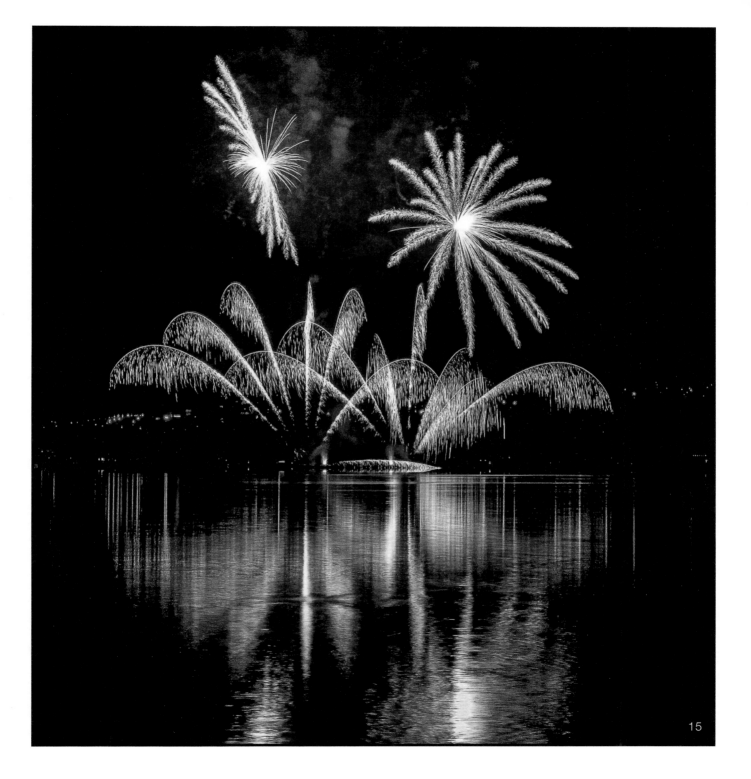

15

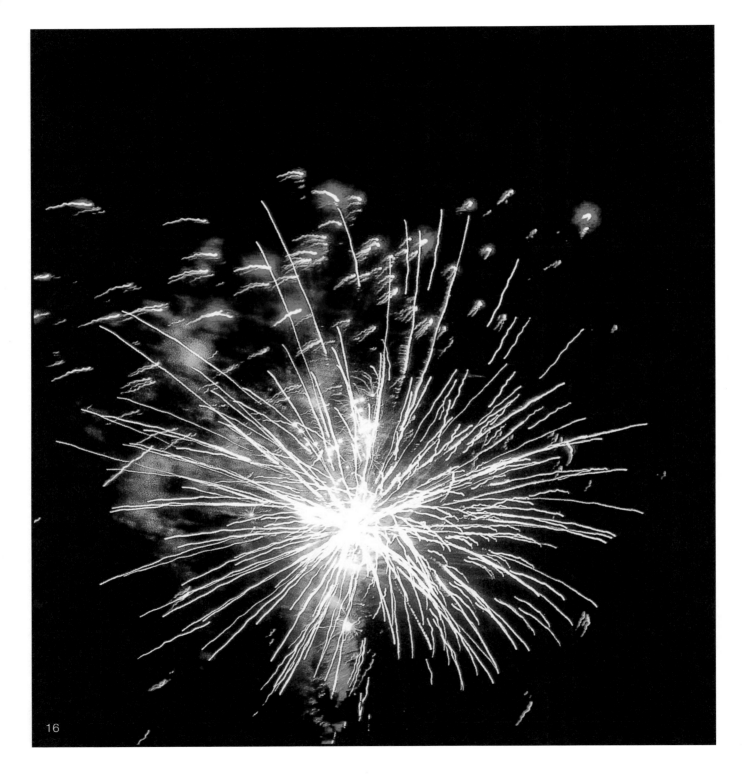

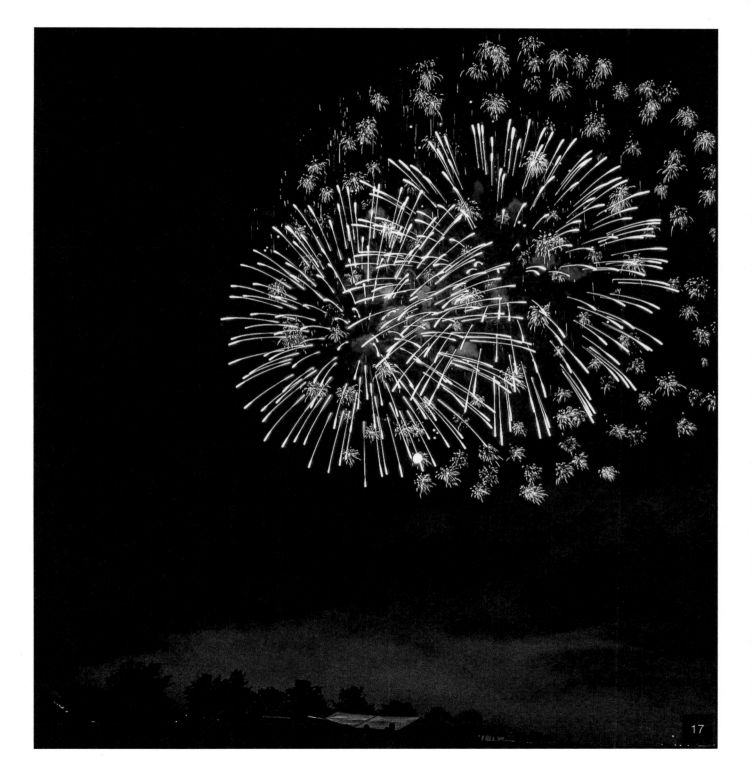

17

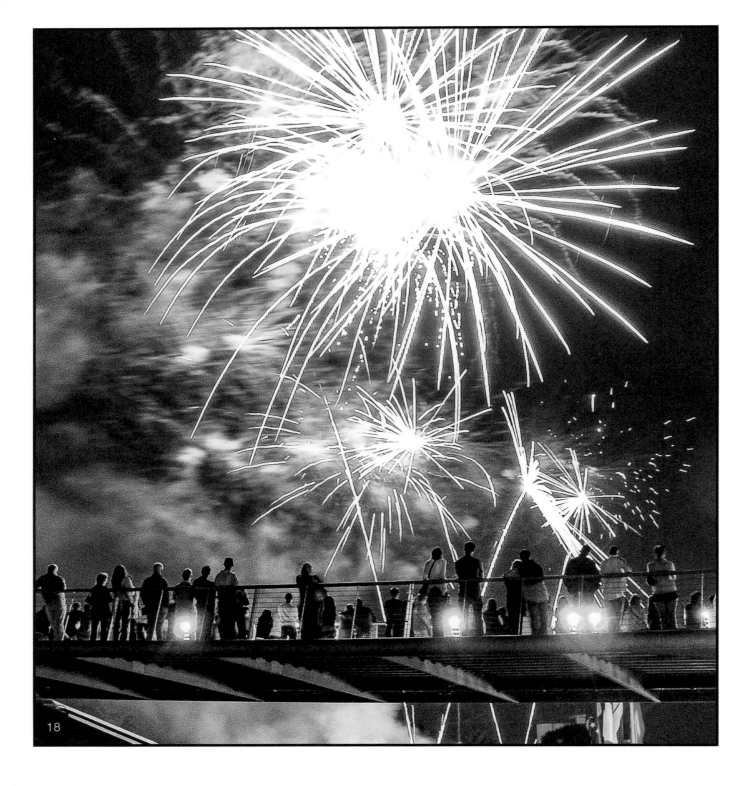

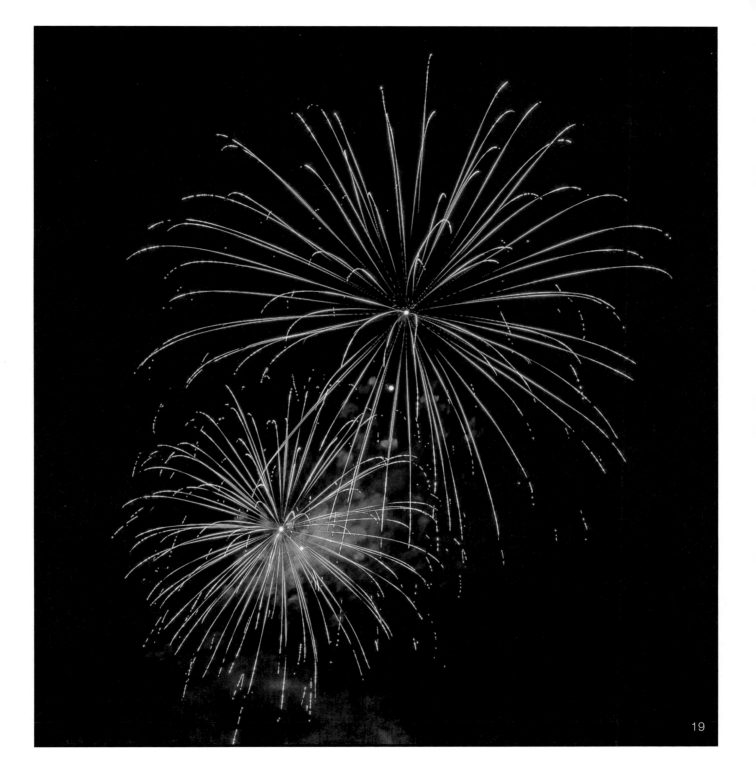

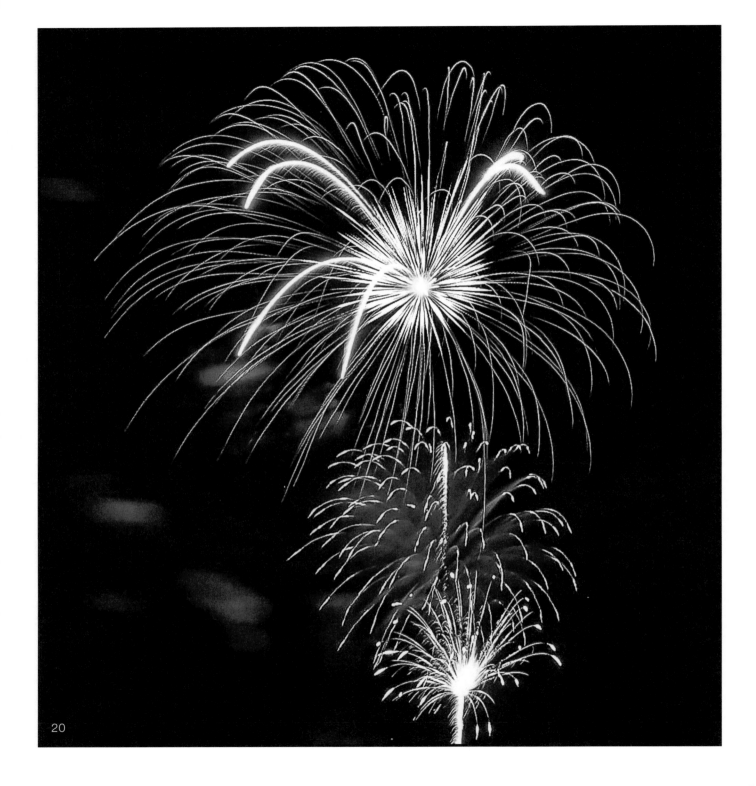

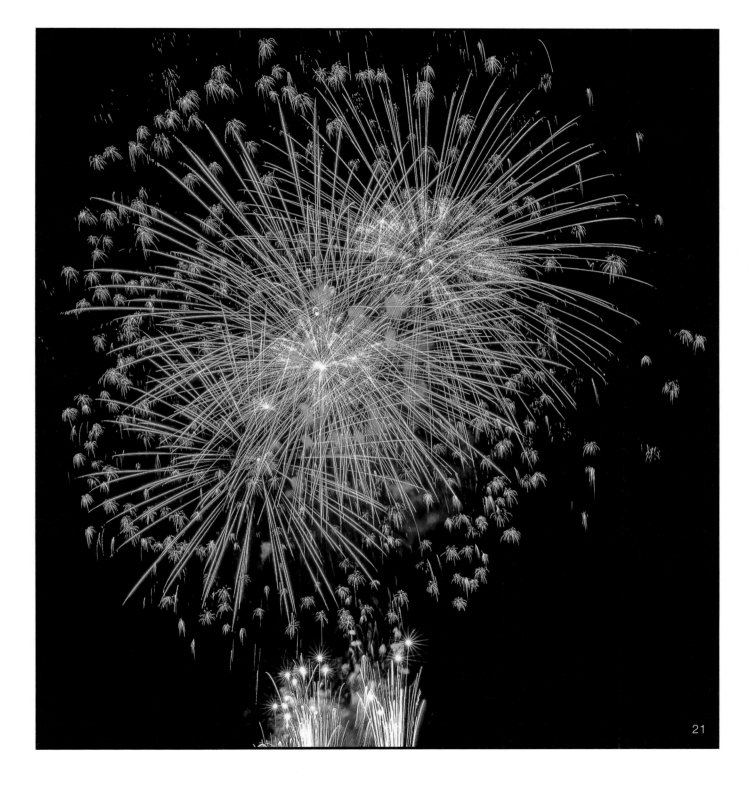

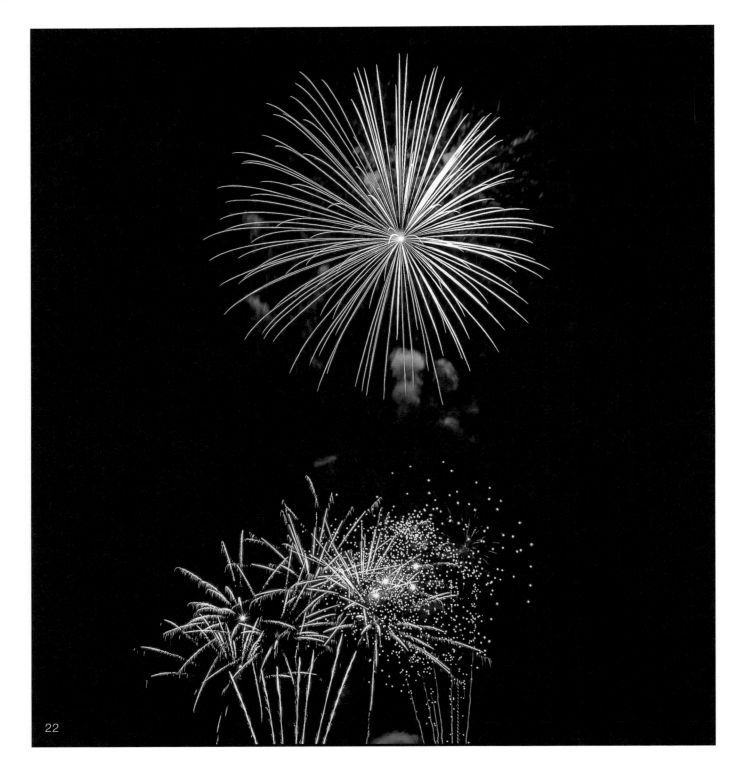

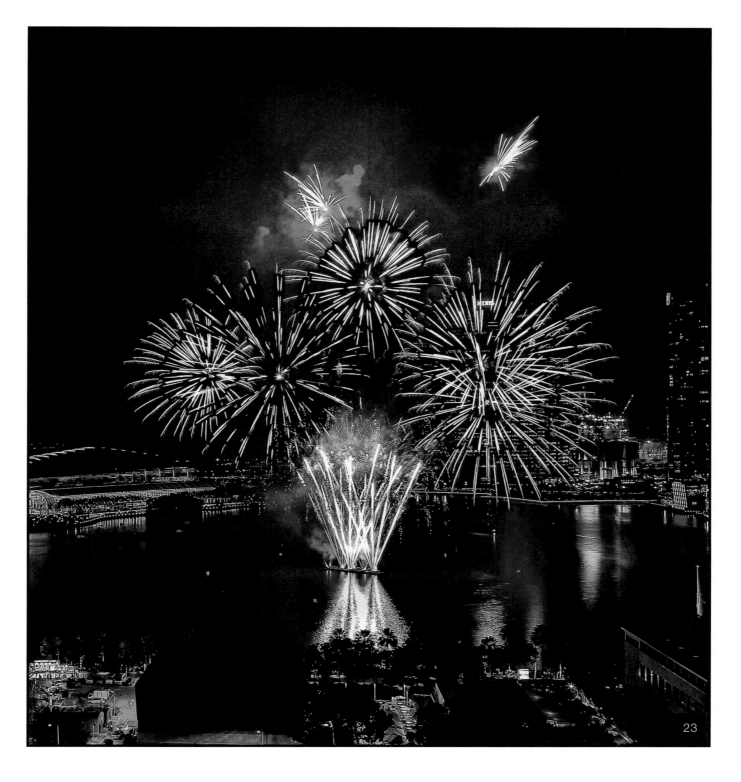

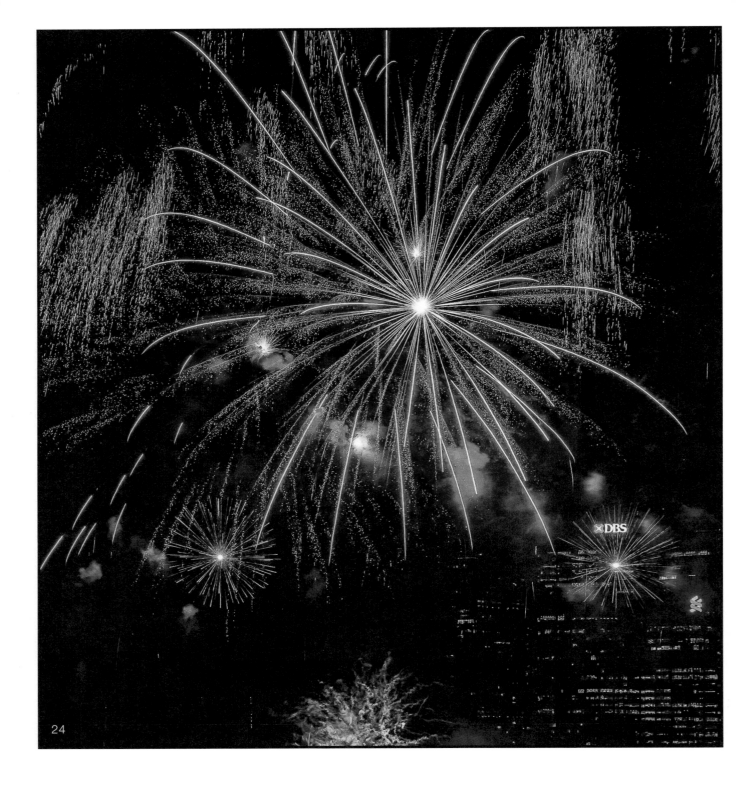

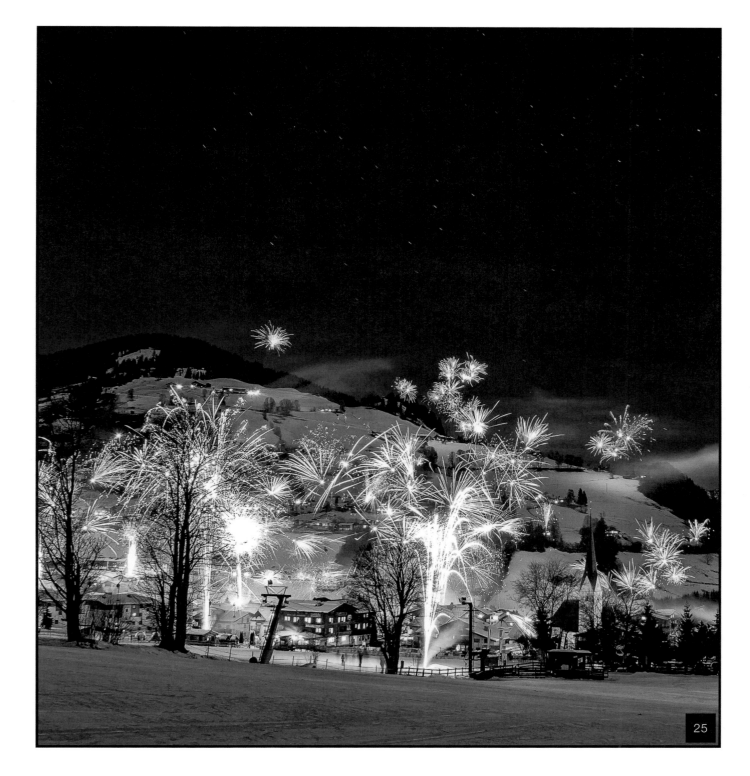

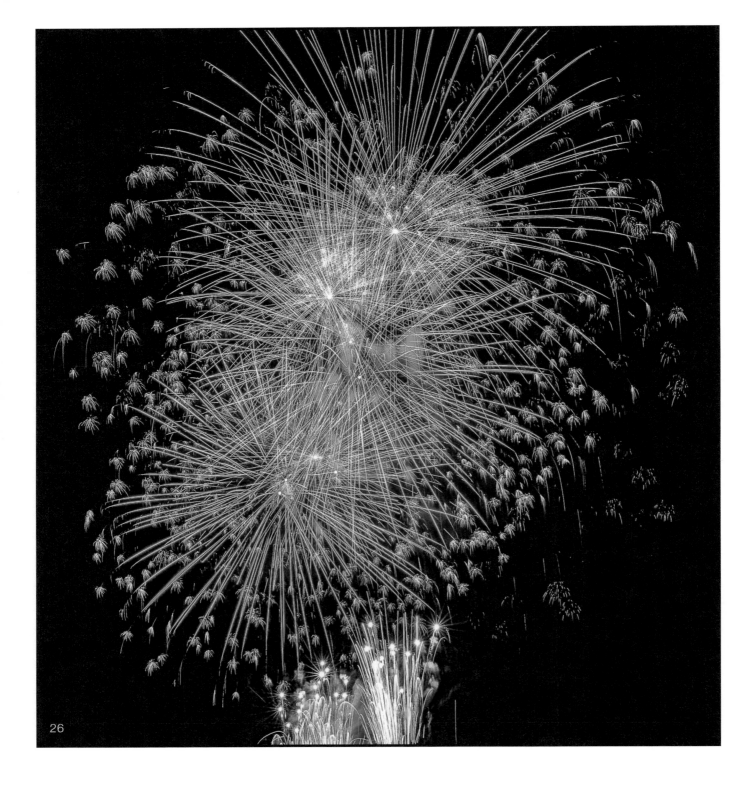

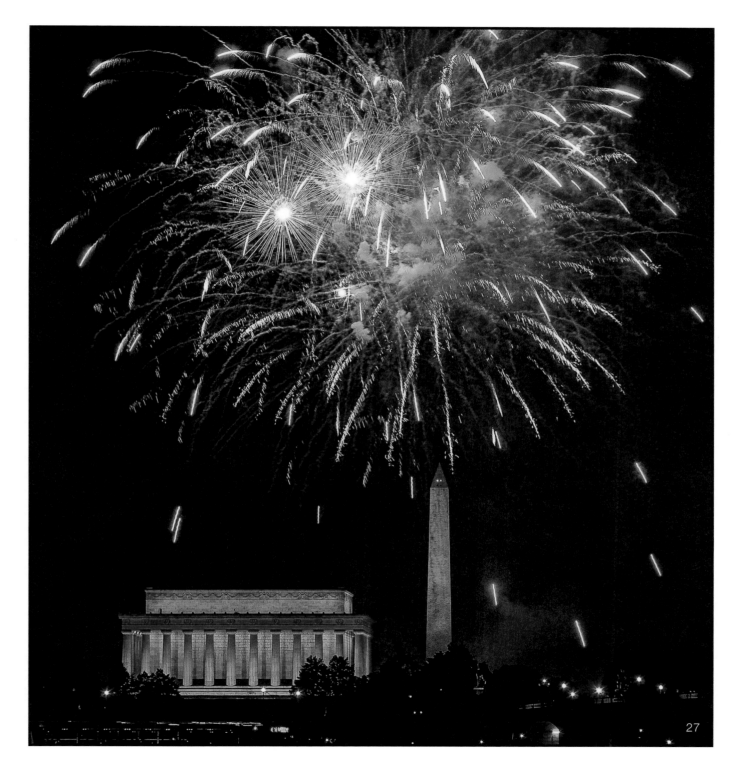

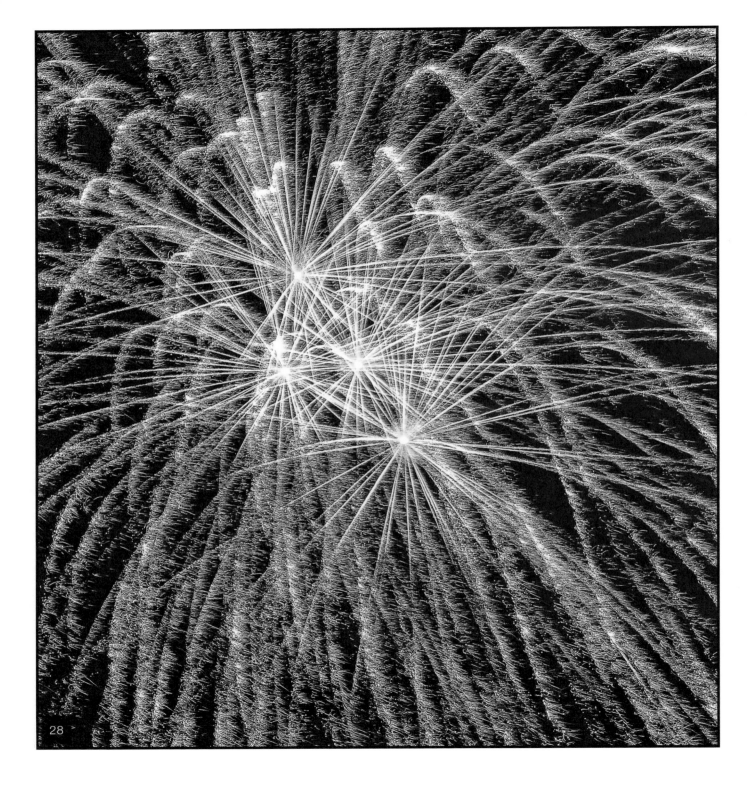

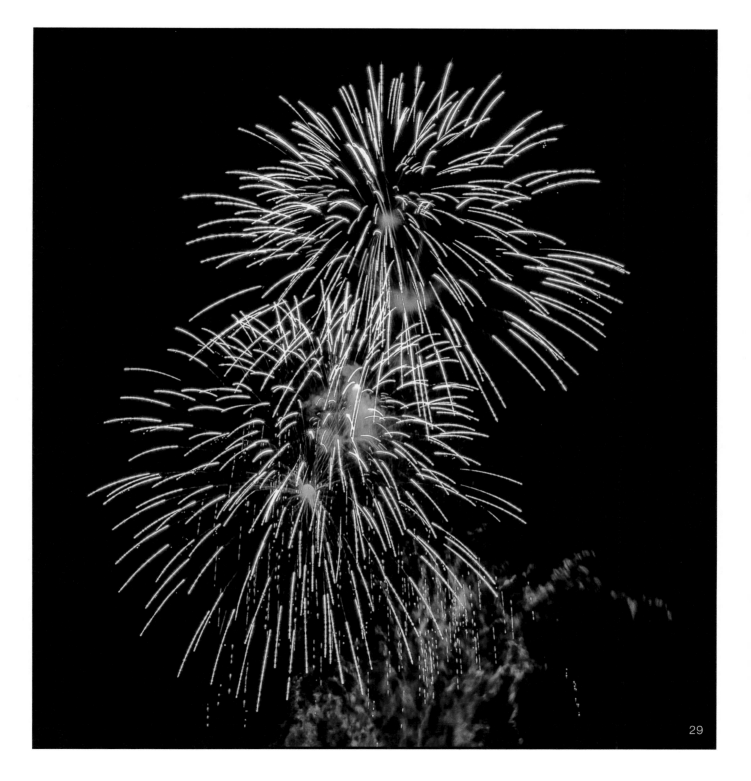

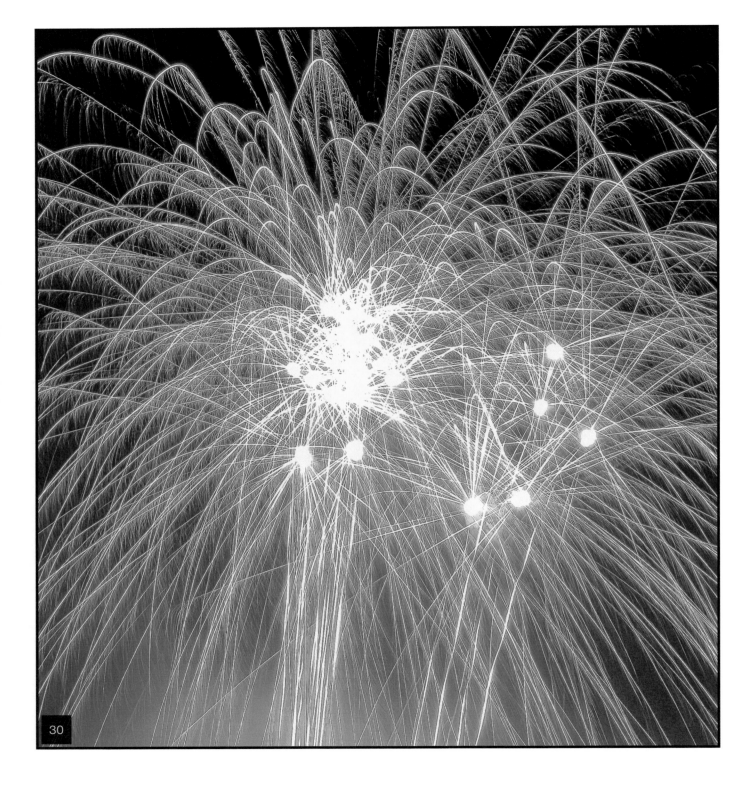

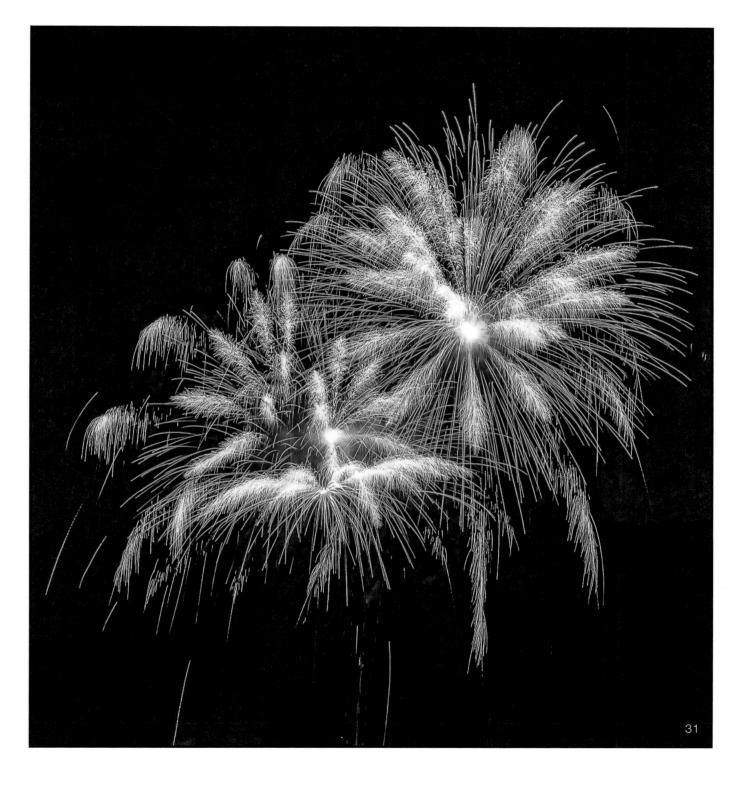

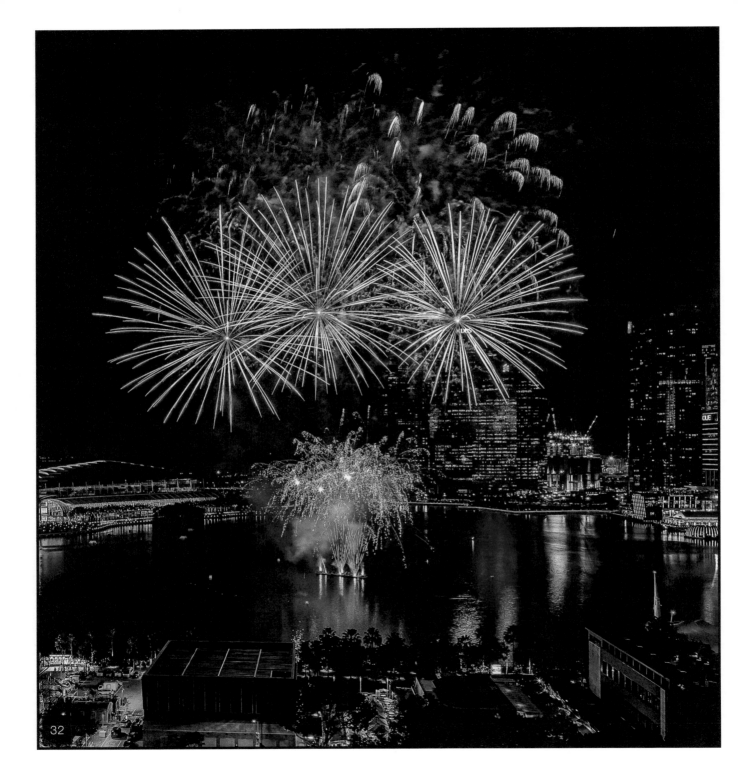

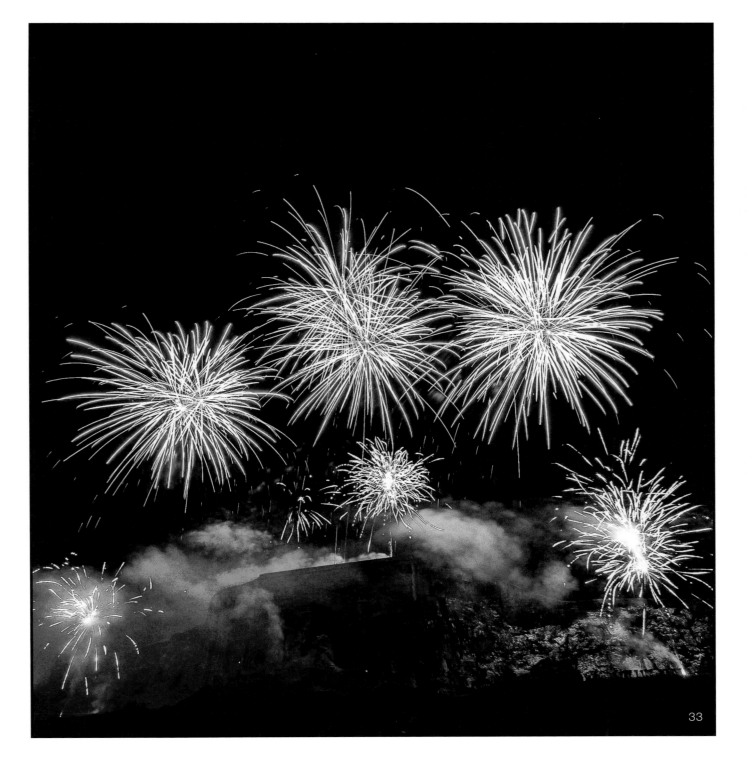

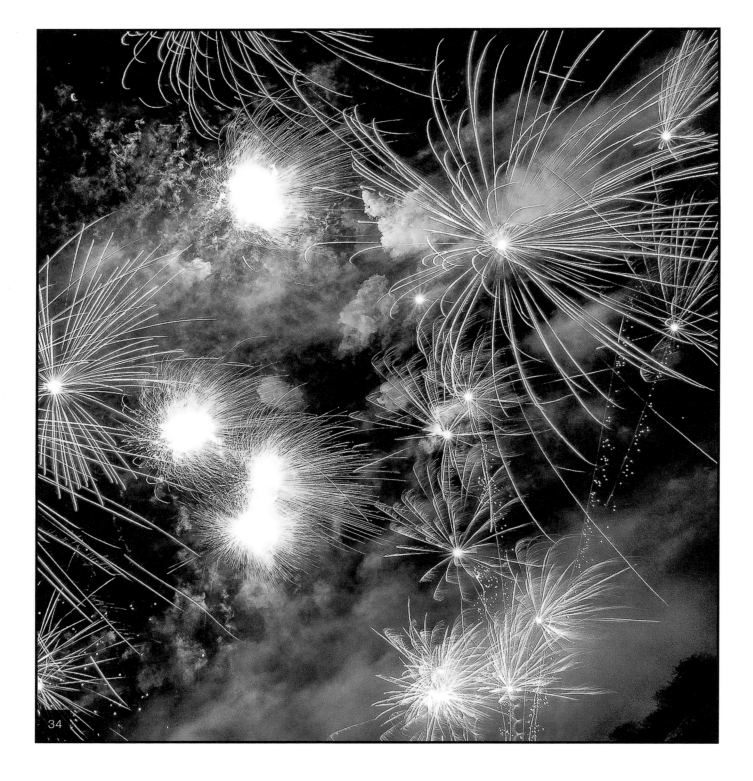

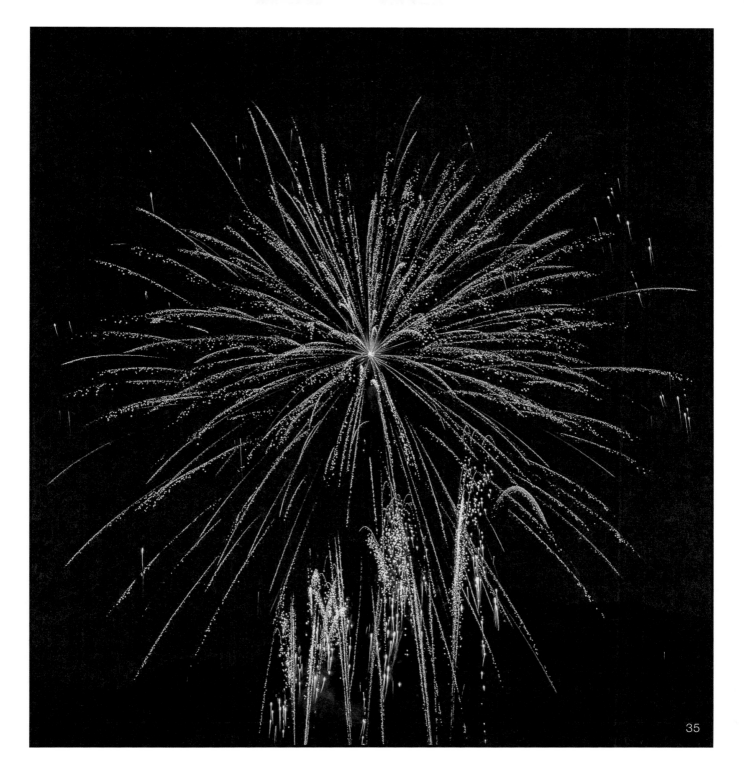

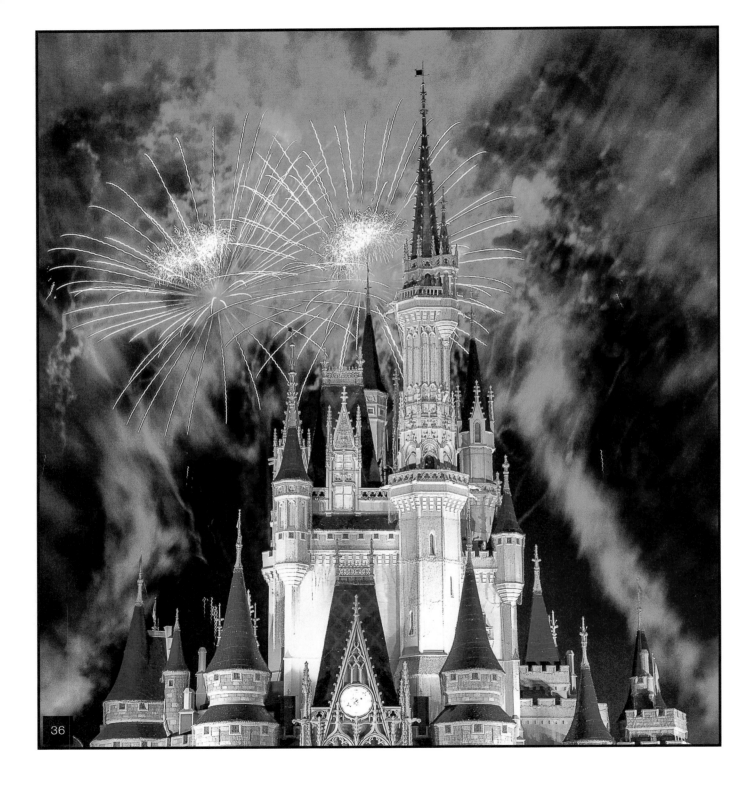

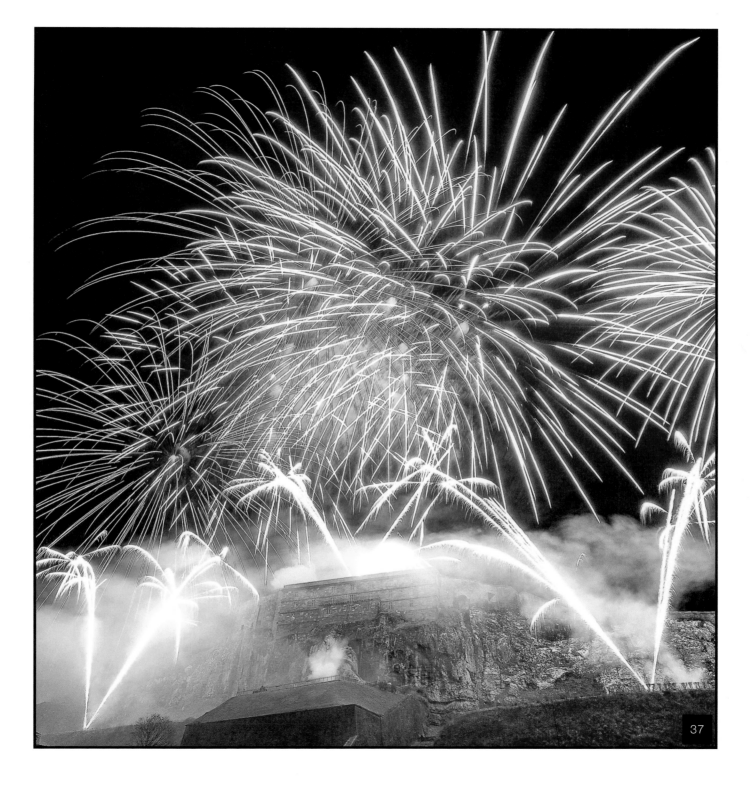

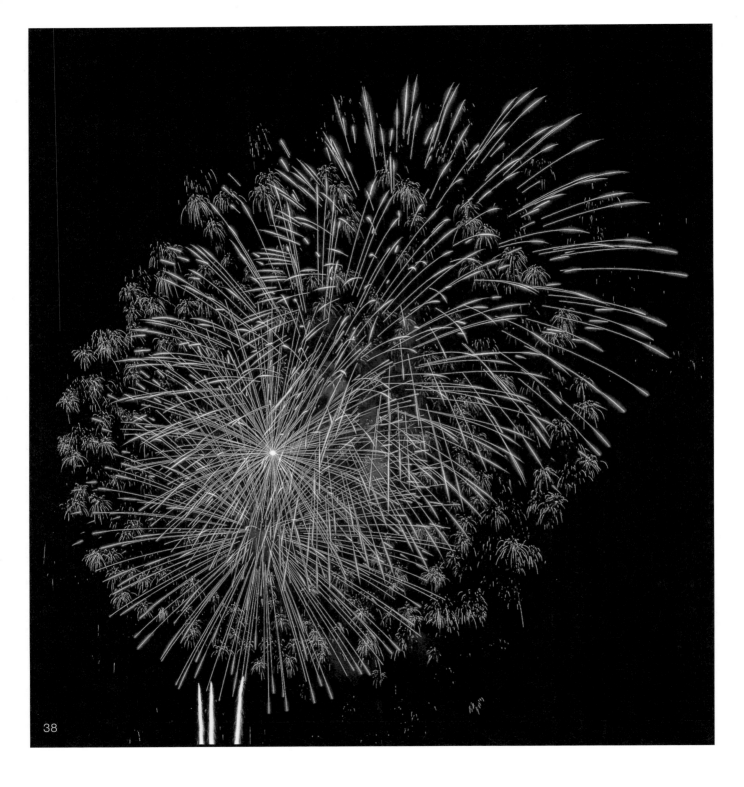

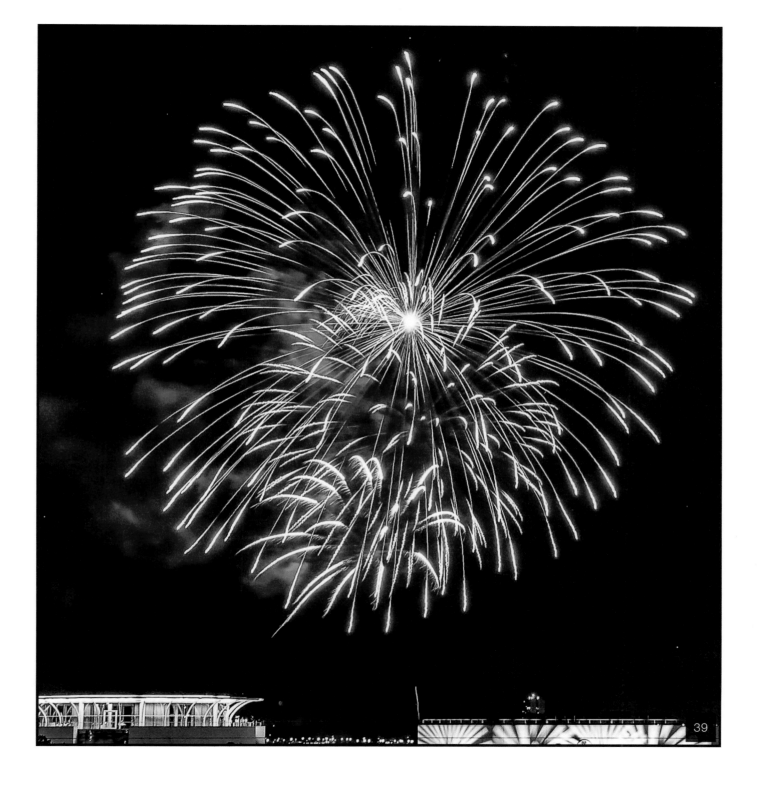

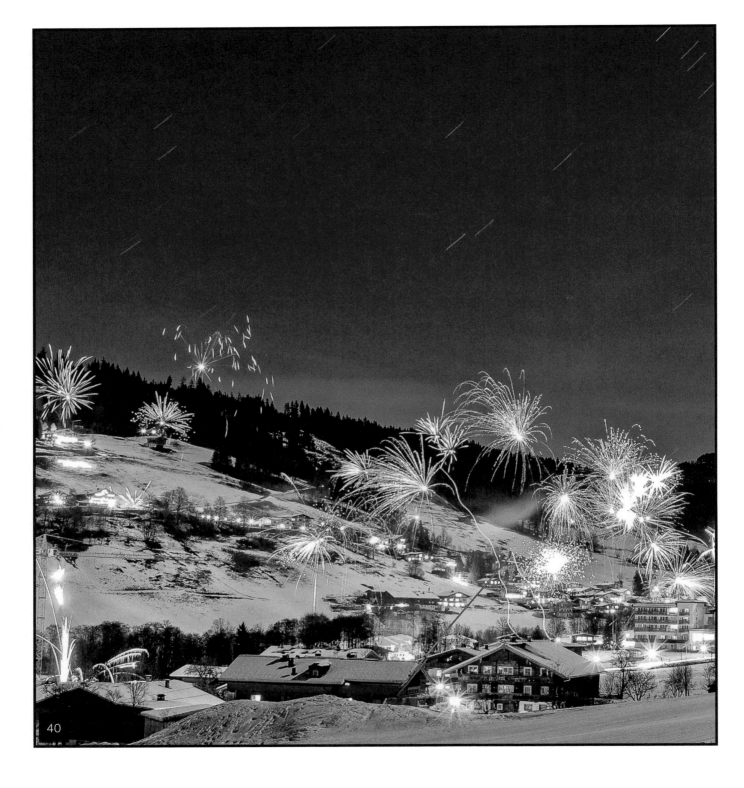

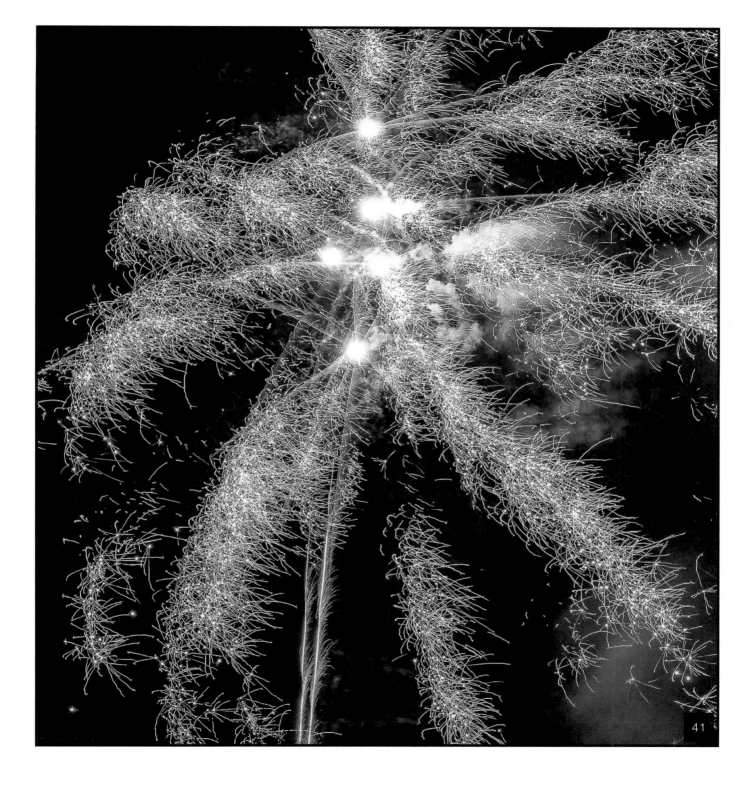

41

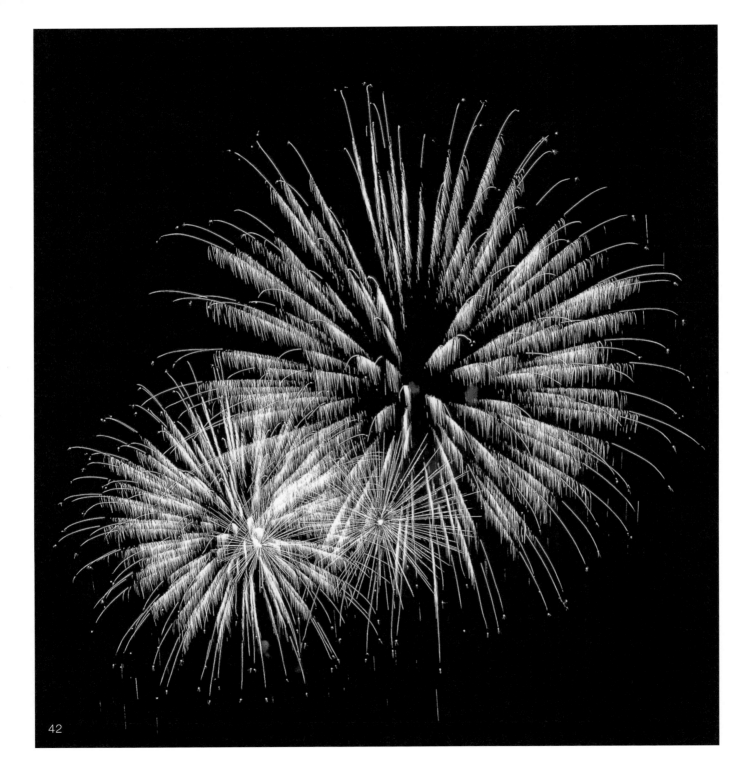

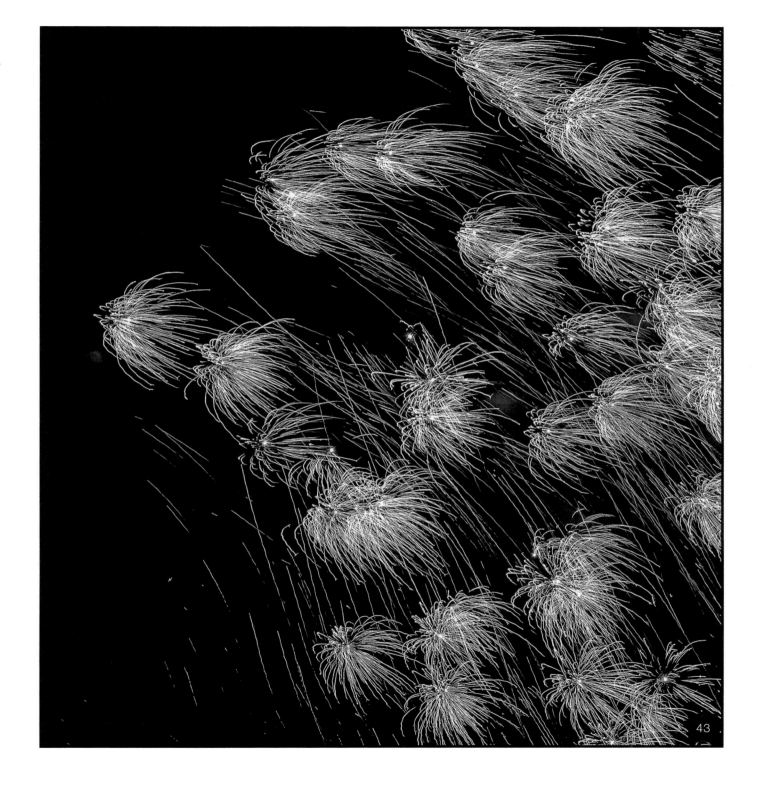

43

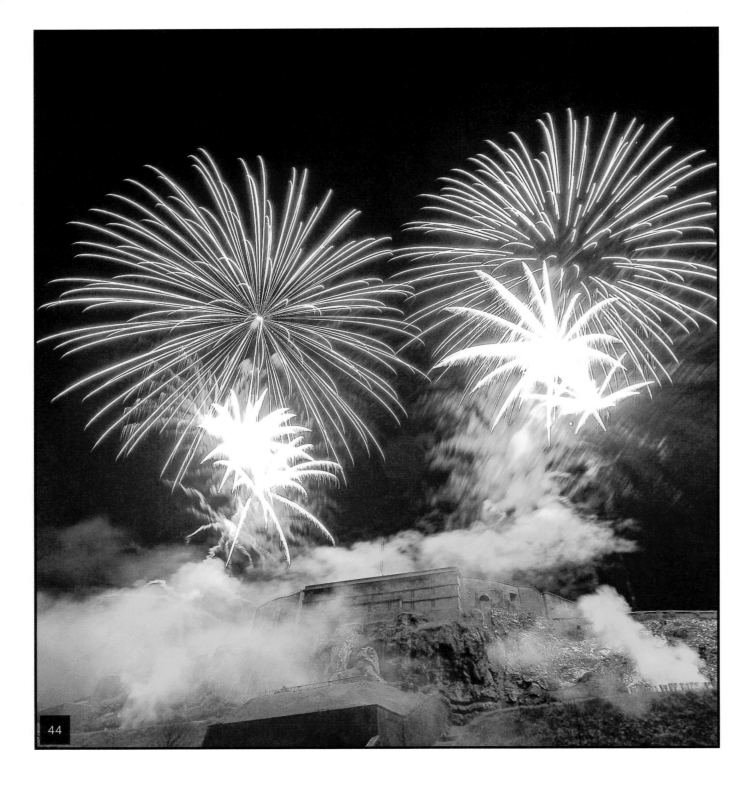

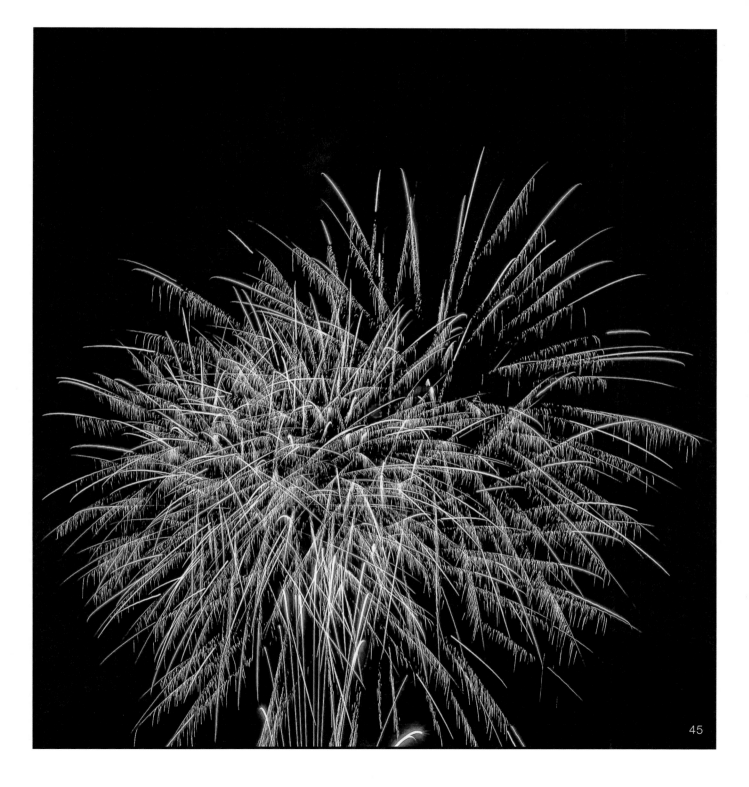

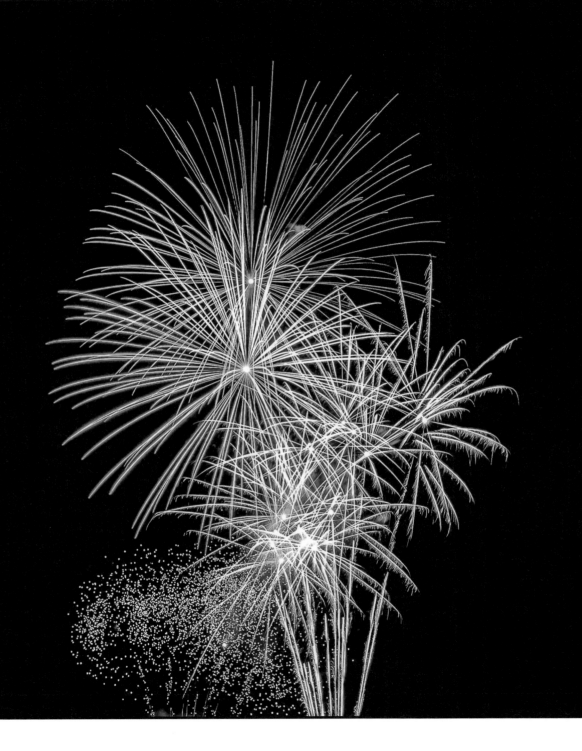

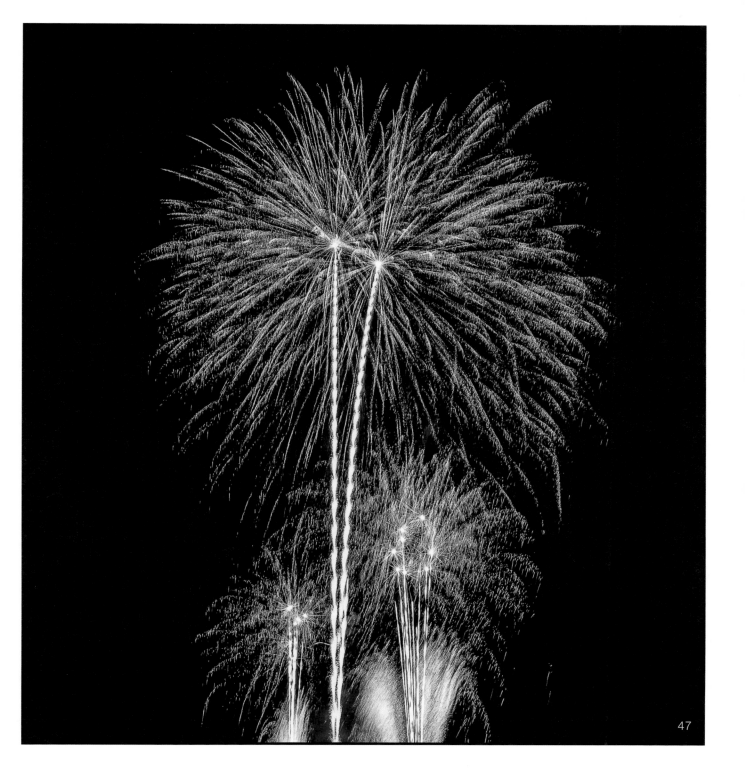

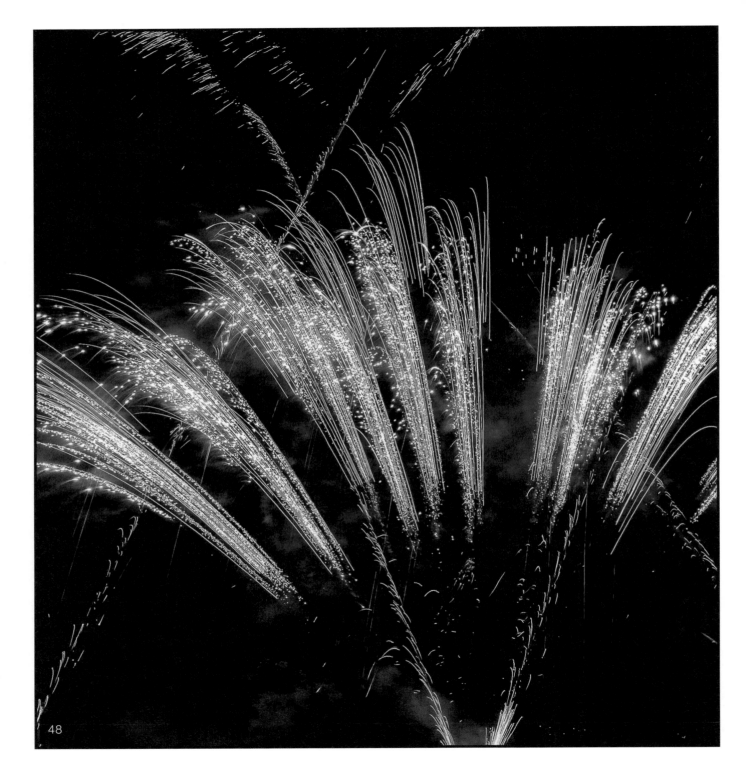
48

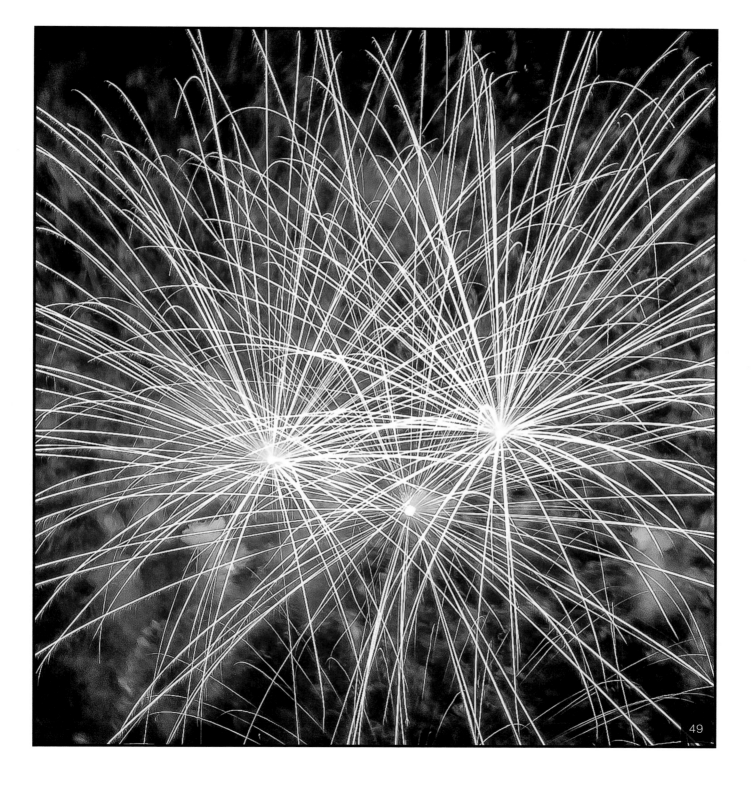

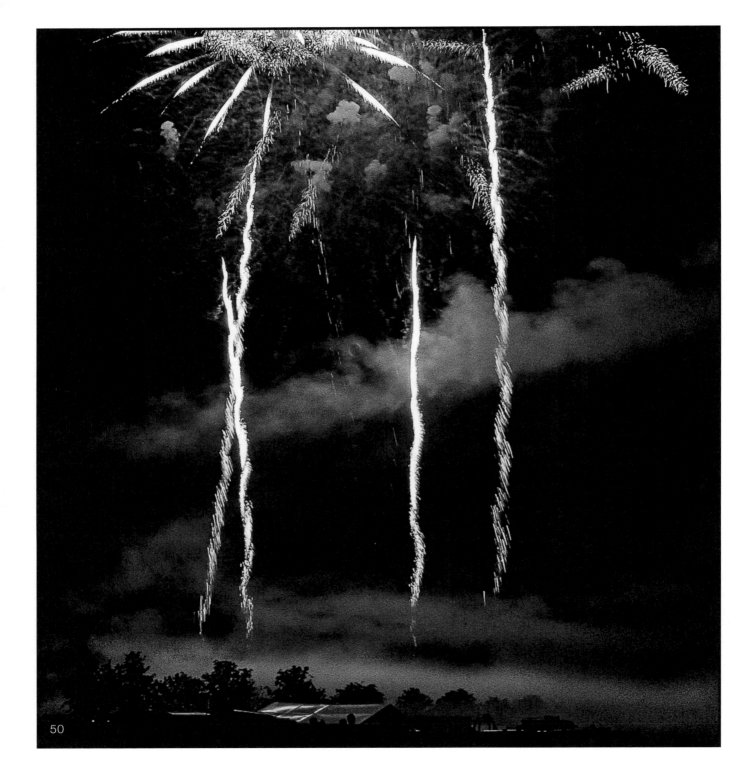

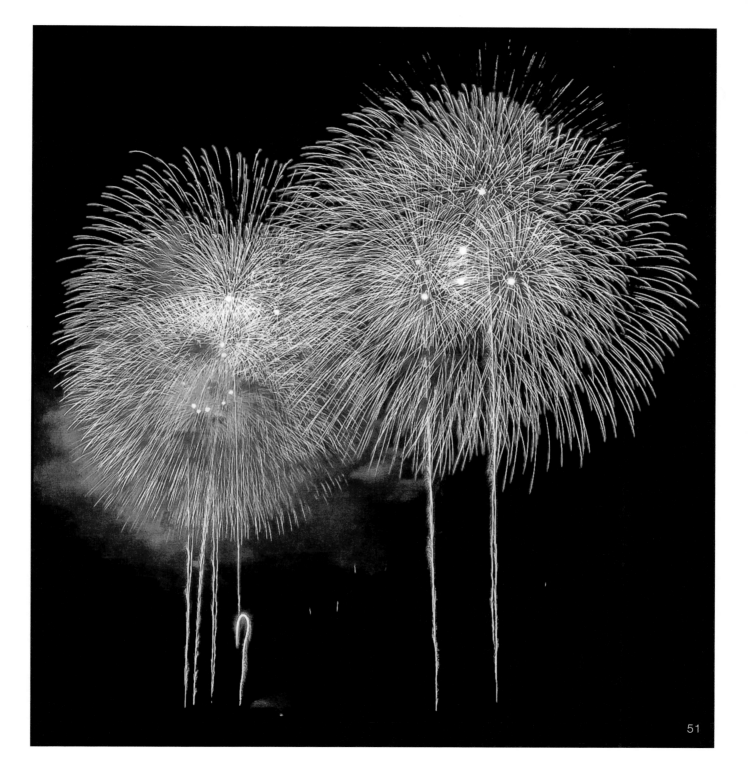

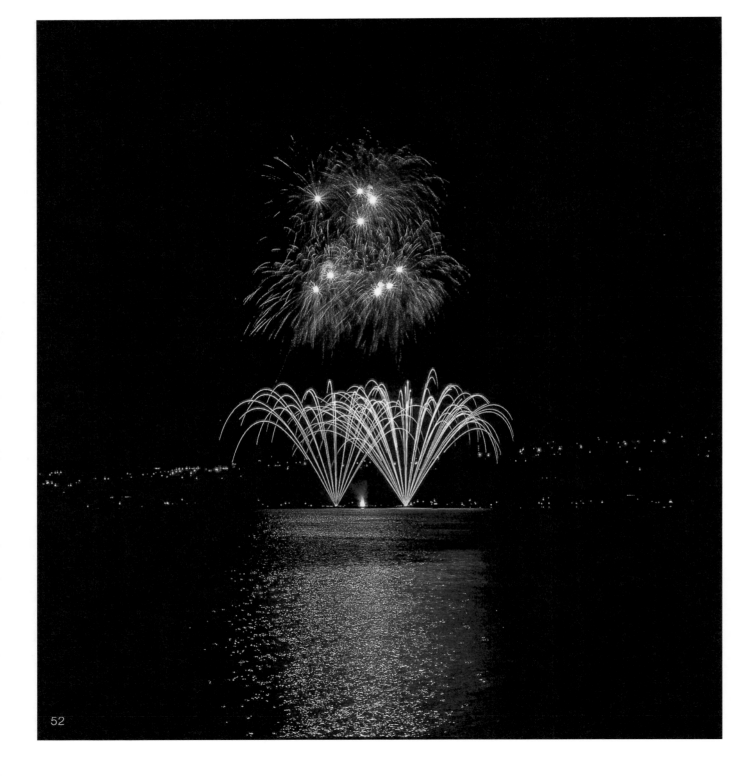

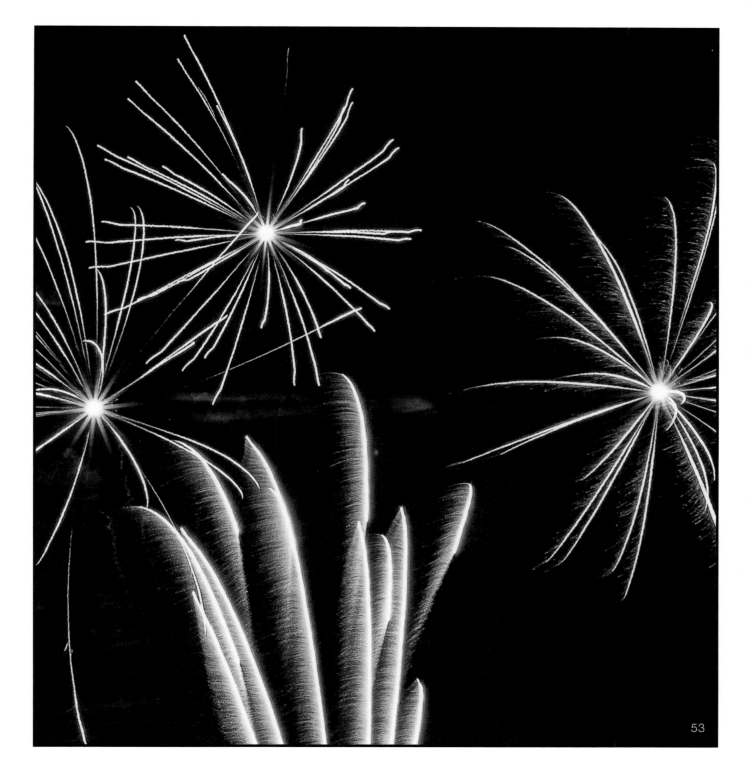

53

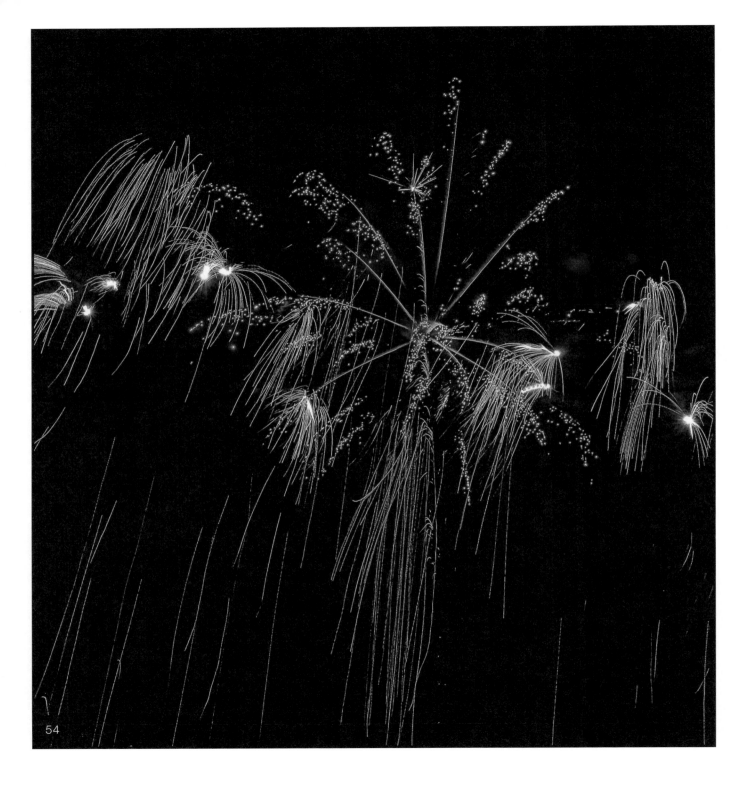

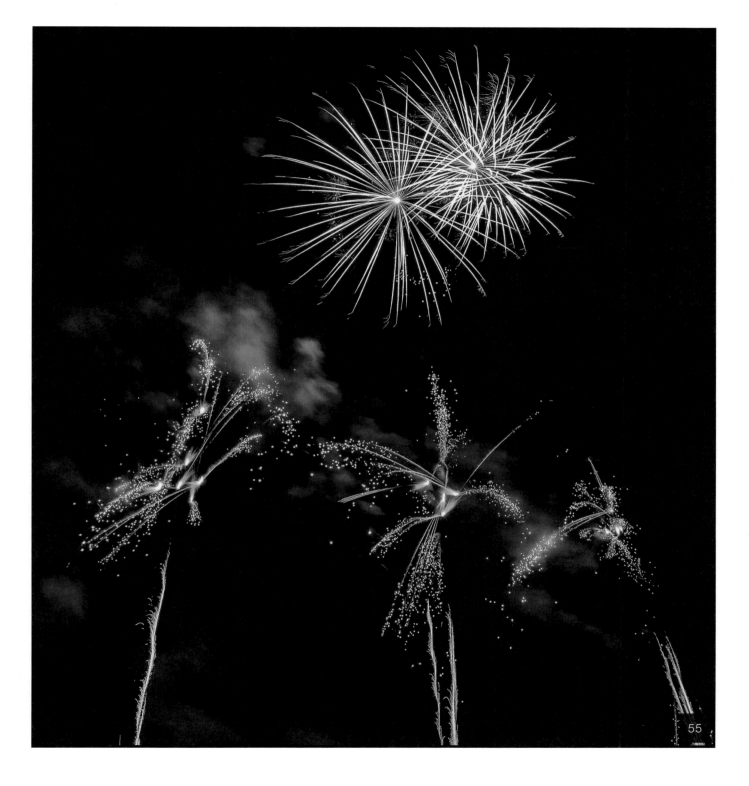

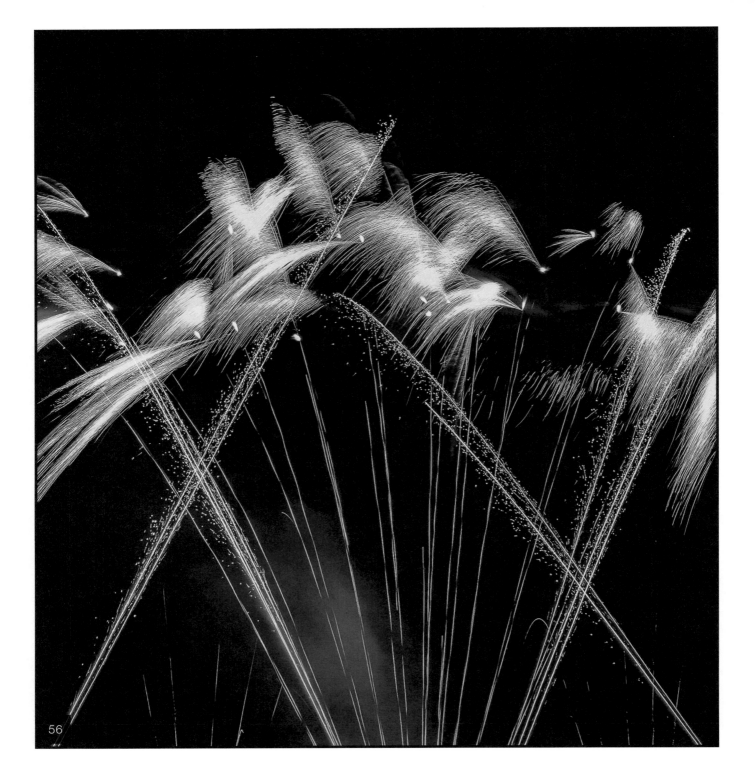

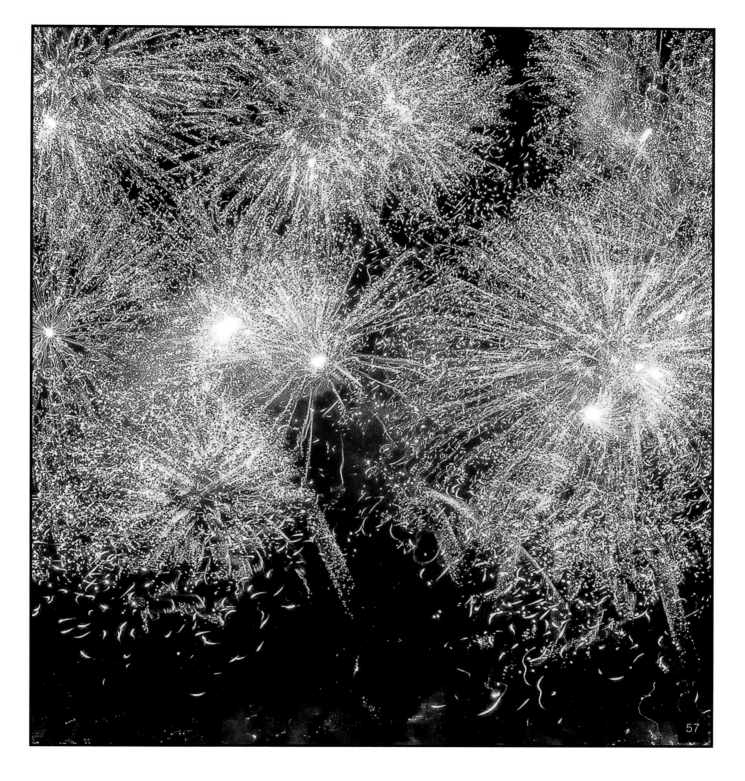

57

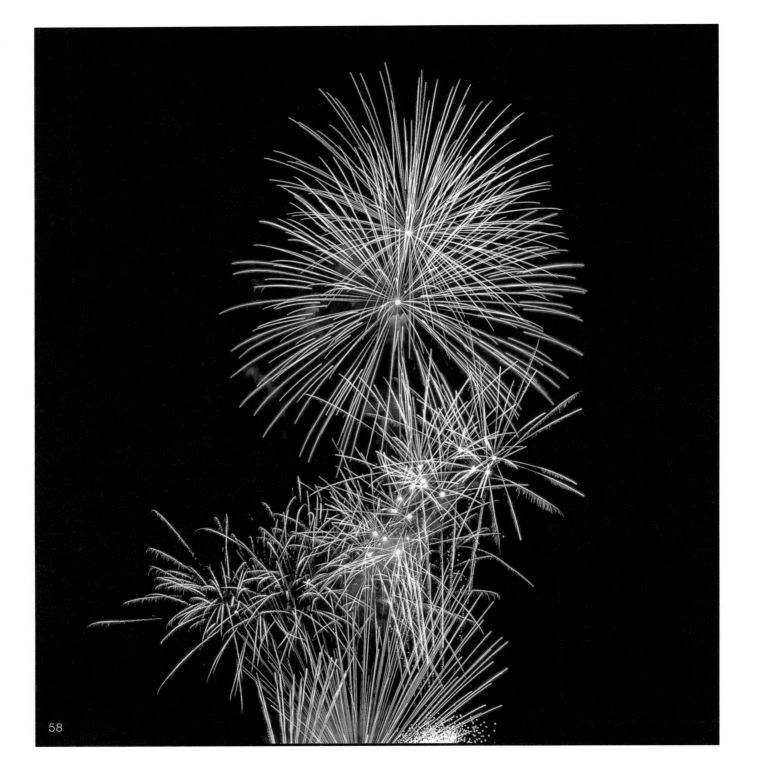

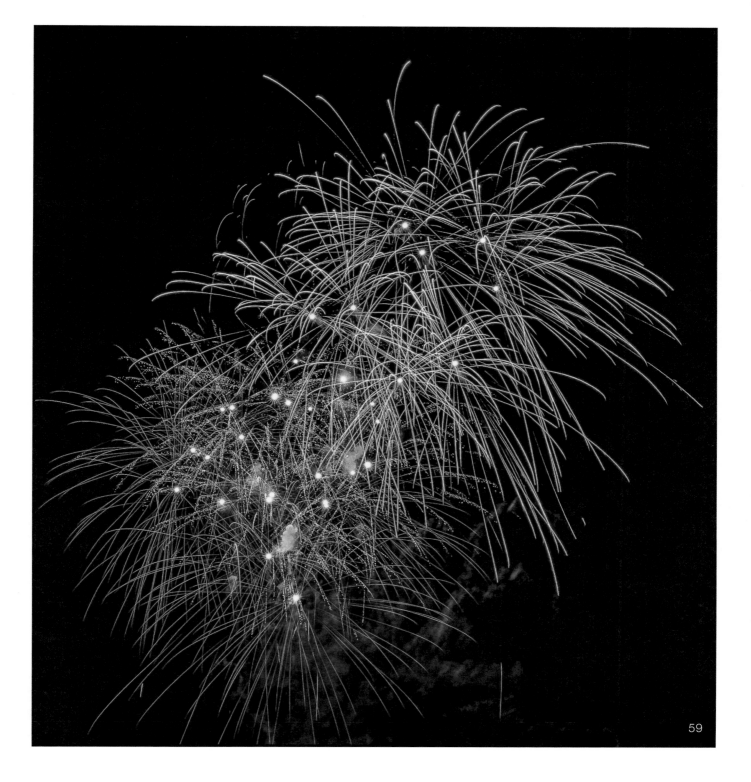

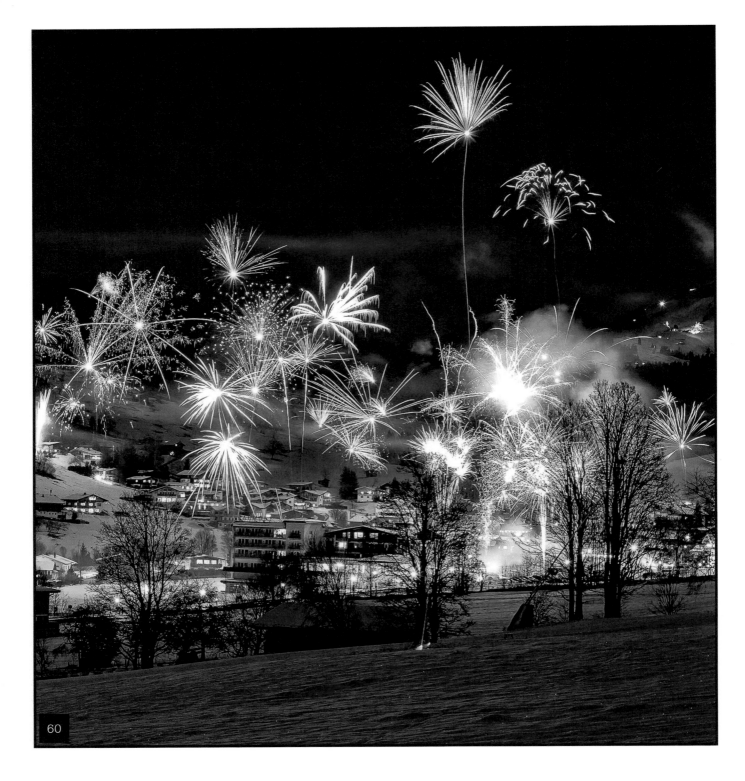

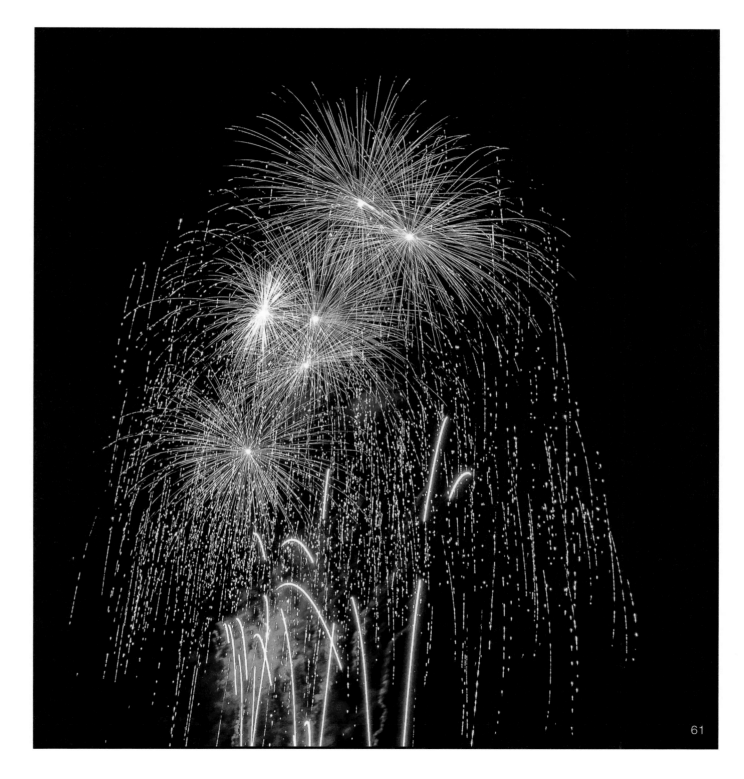

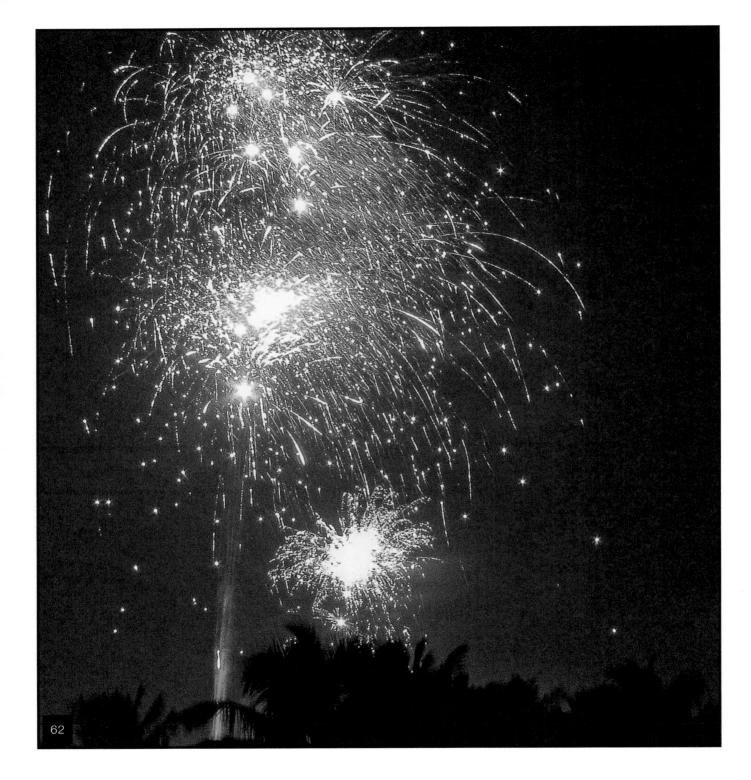

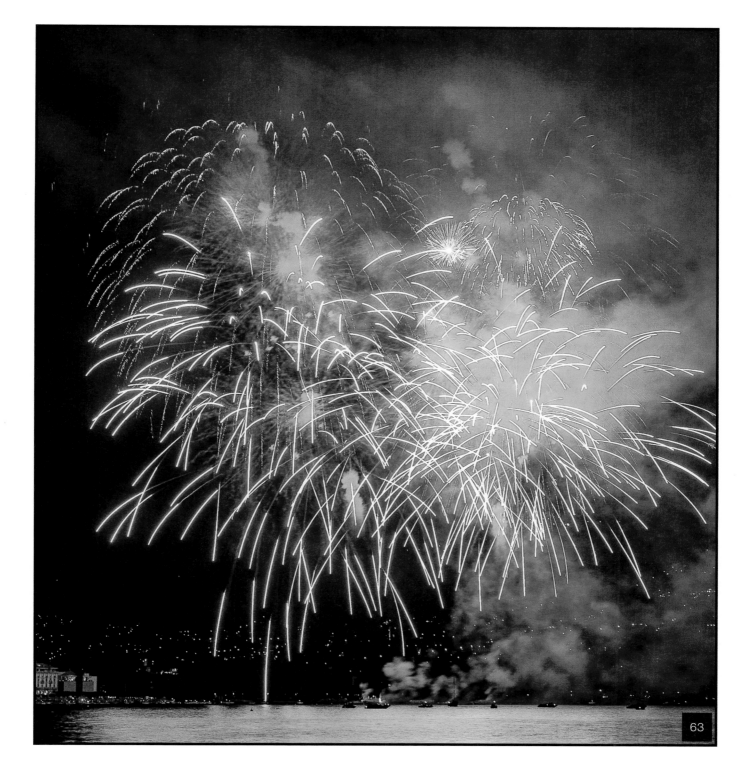

63

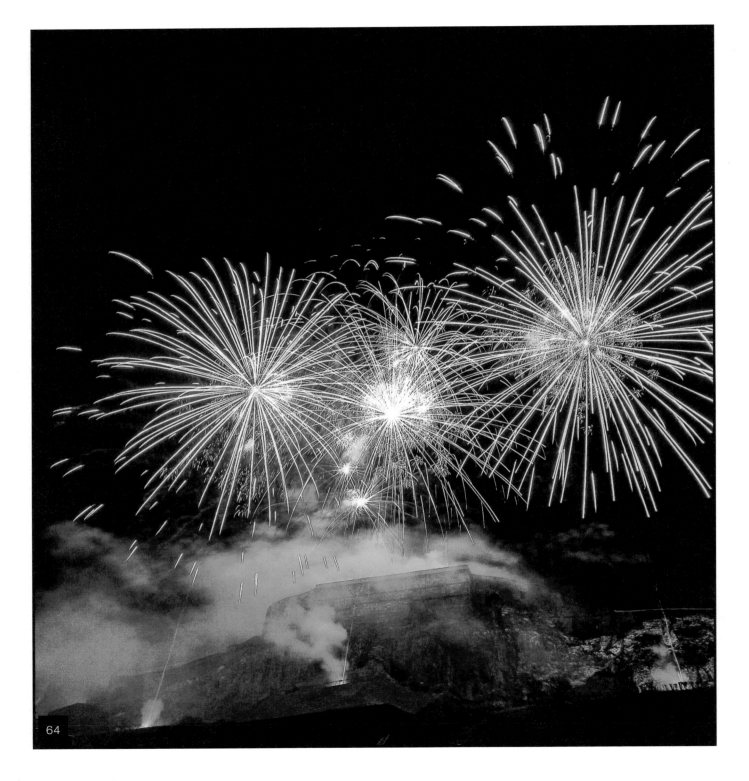

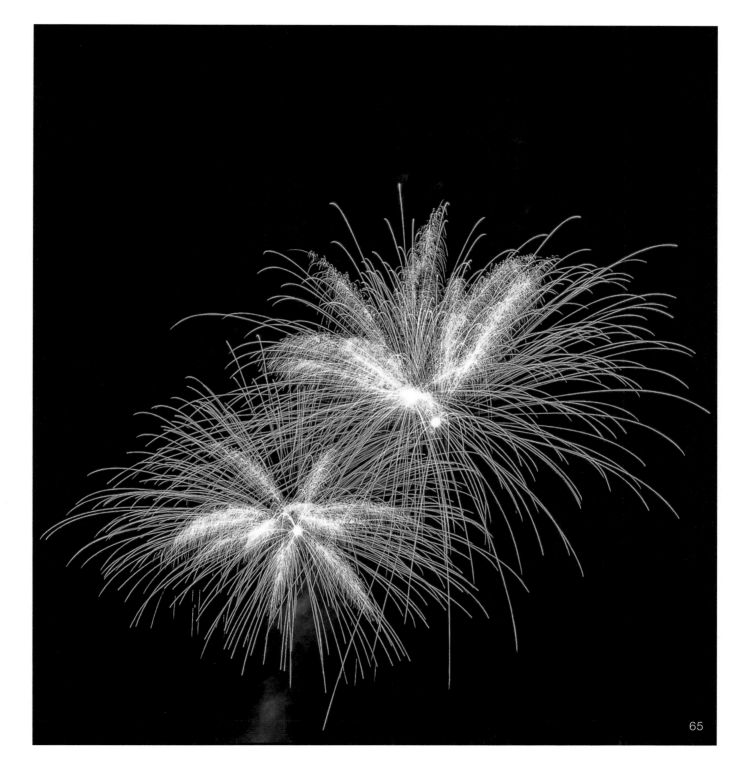

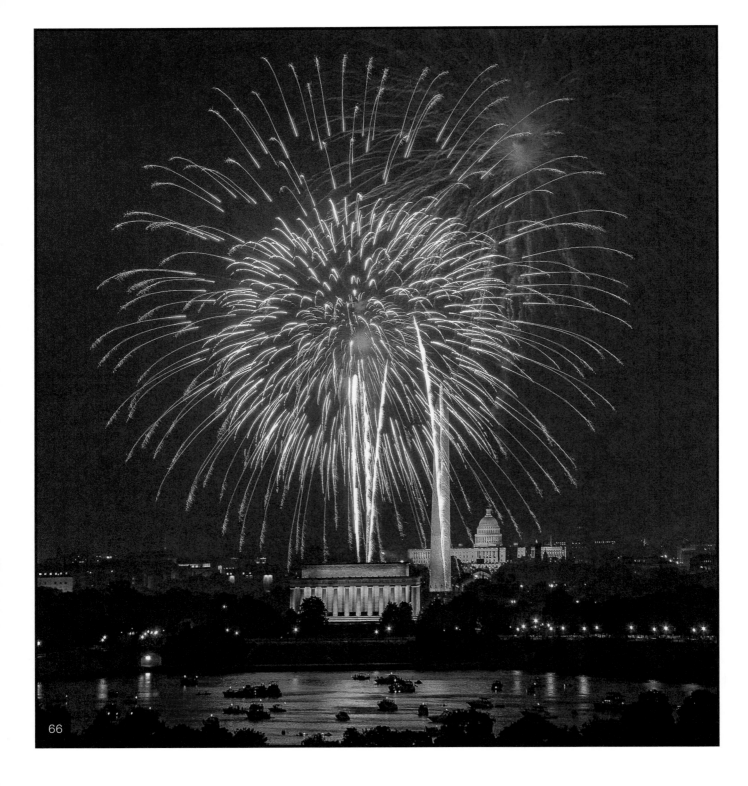

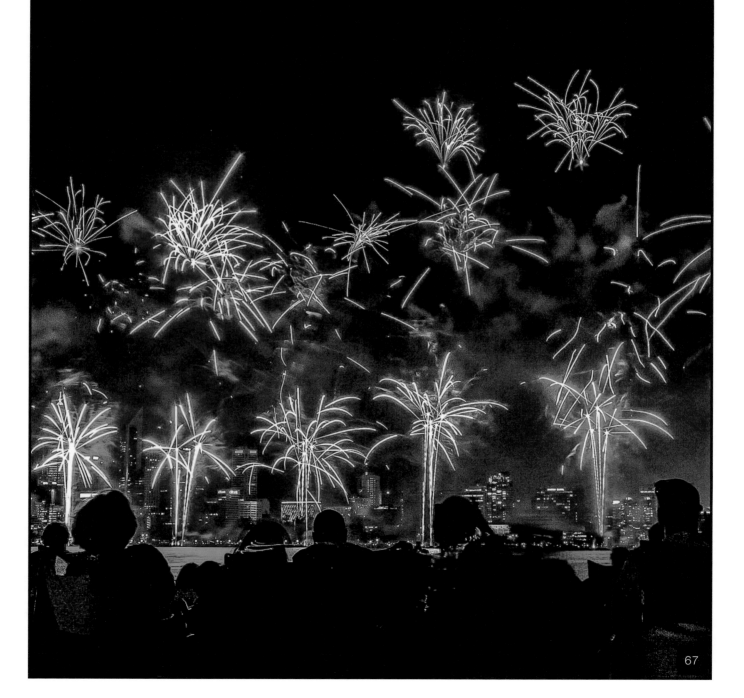

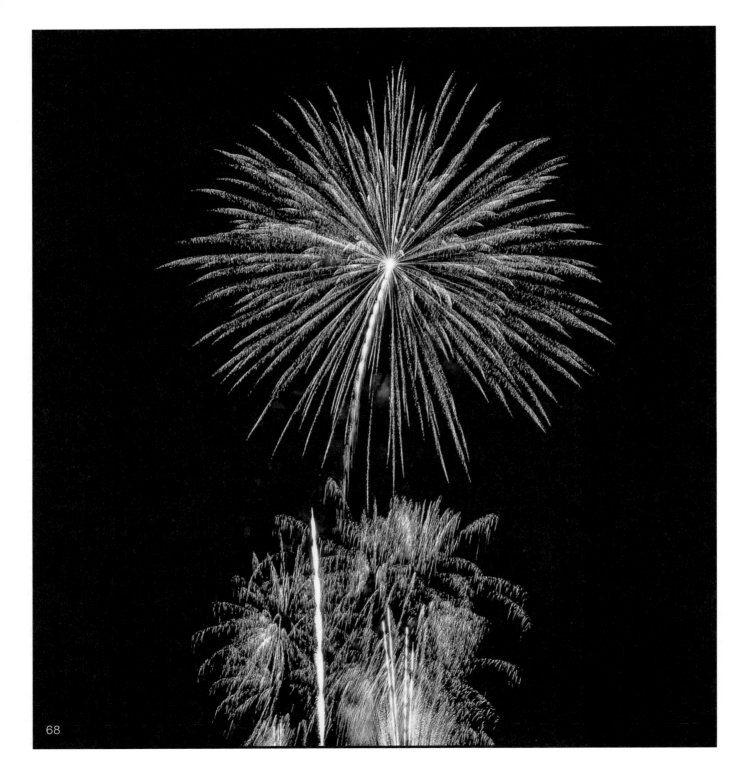

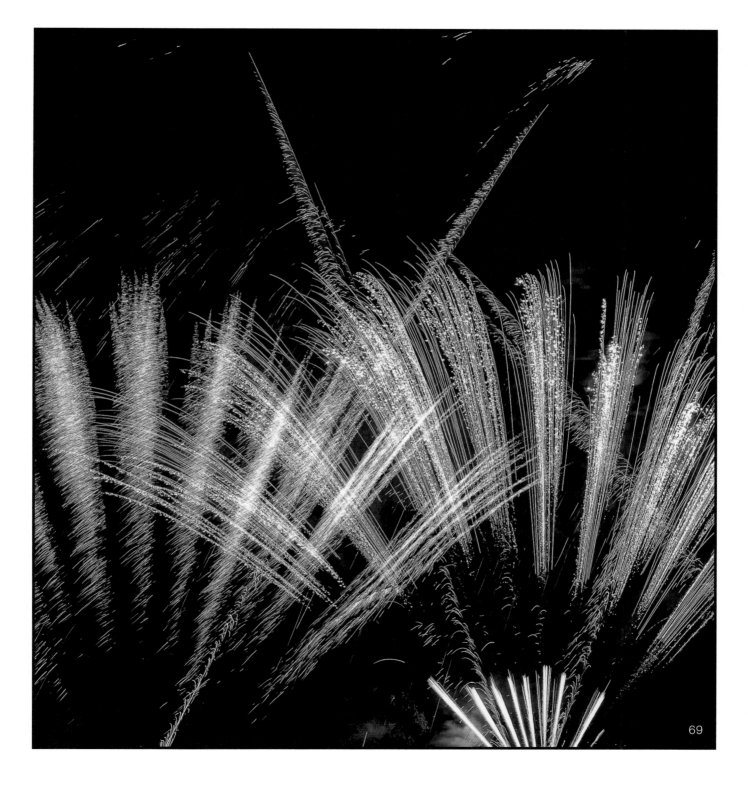

69

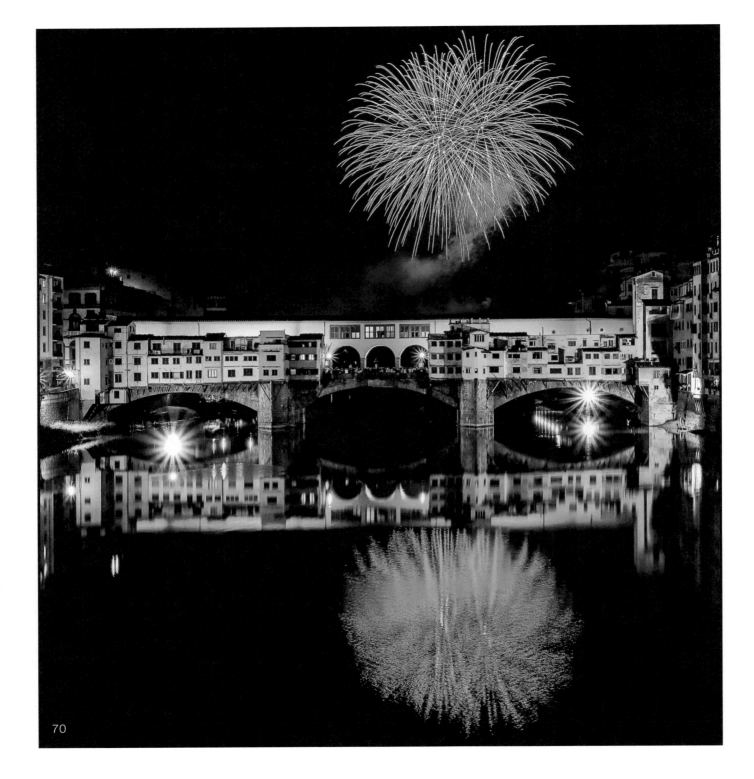

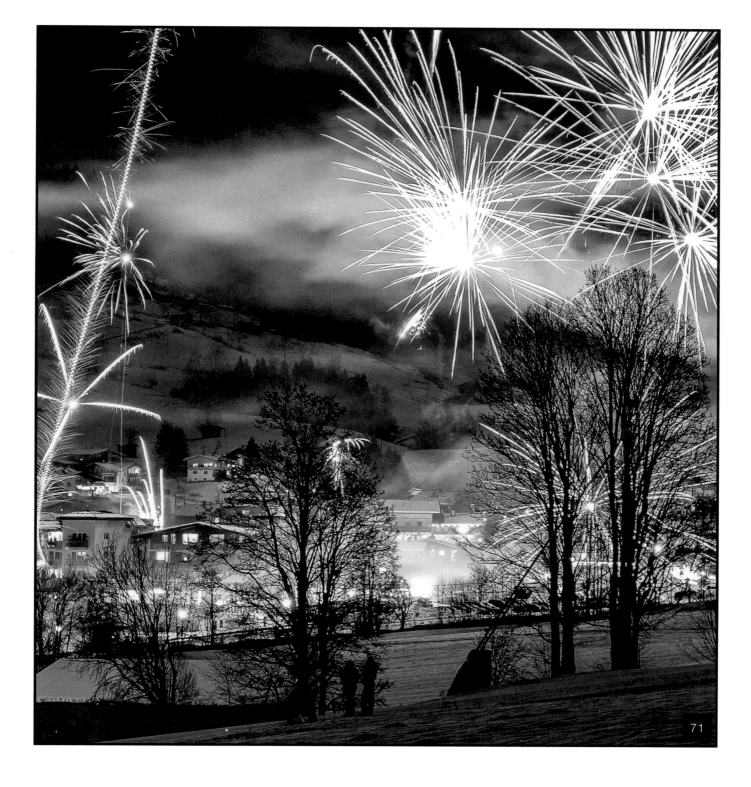

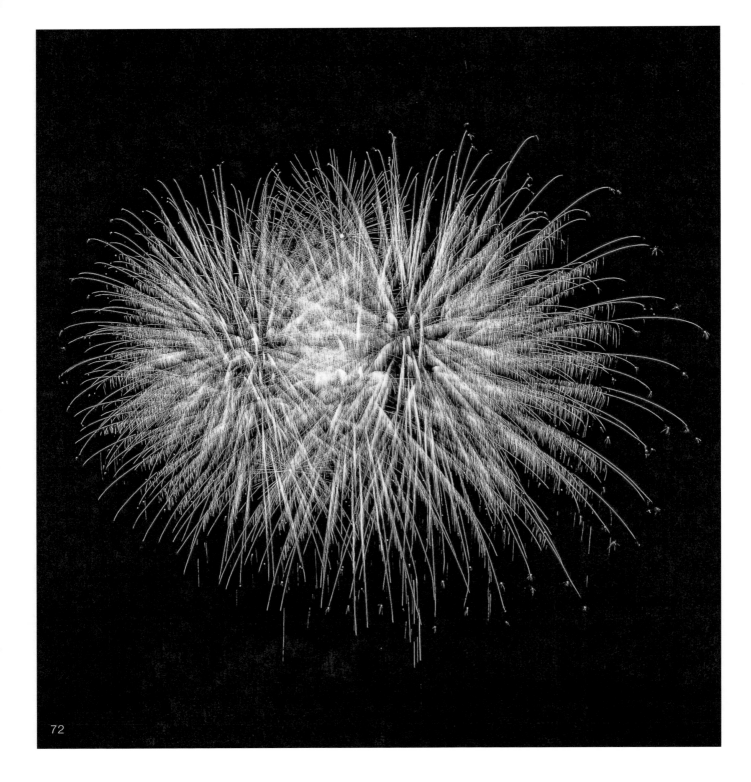

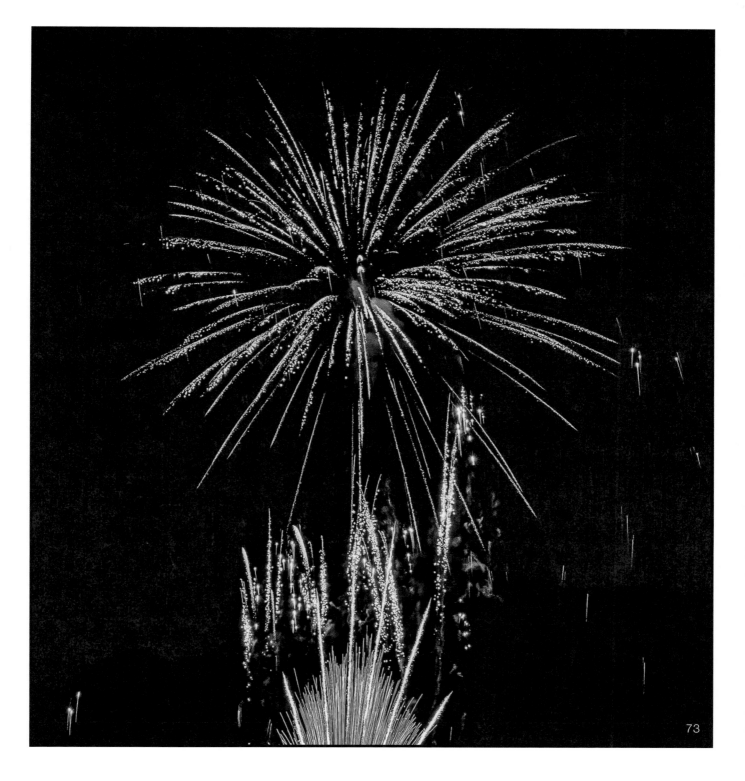

73

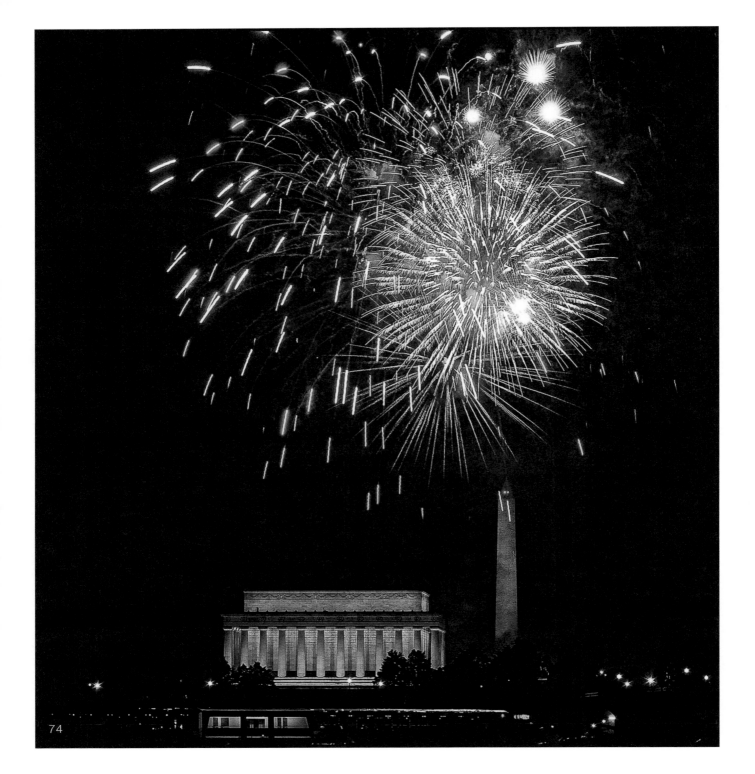

74

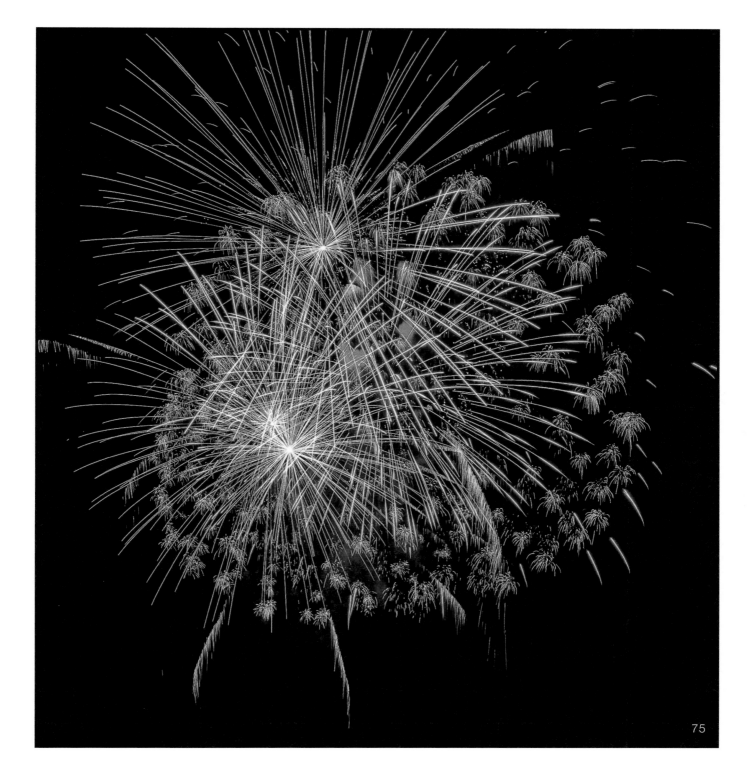

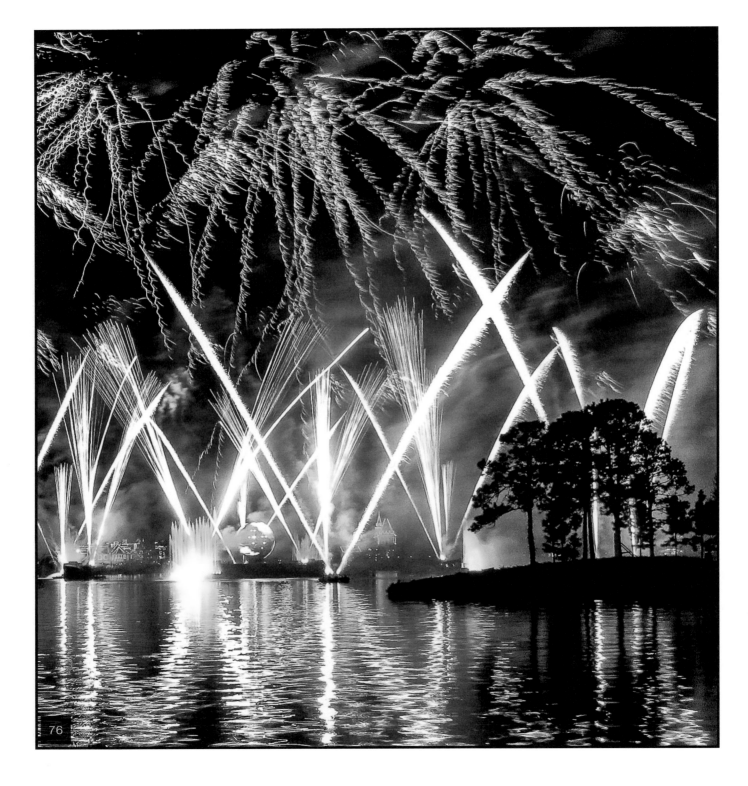

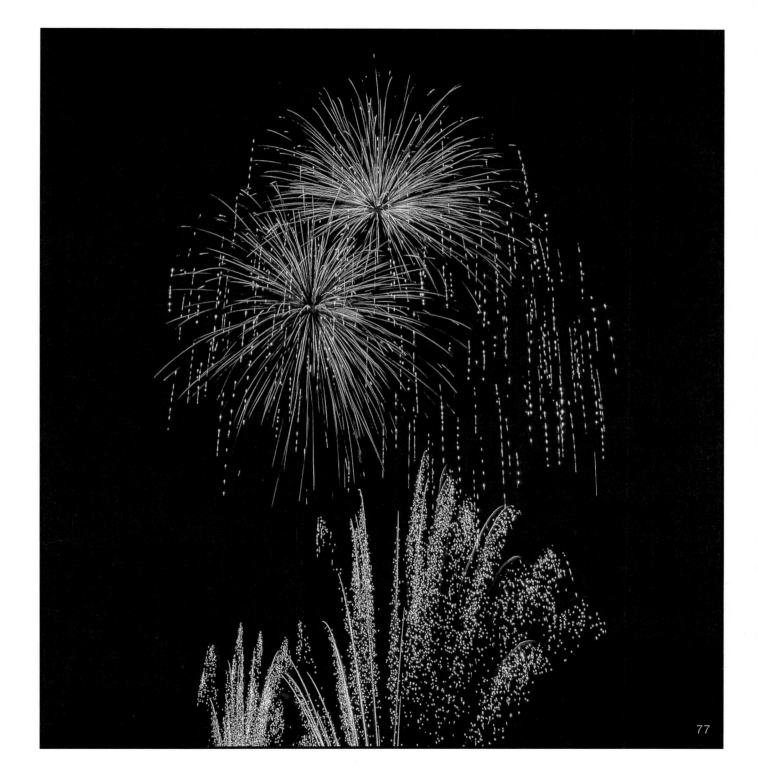

77

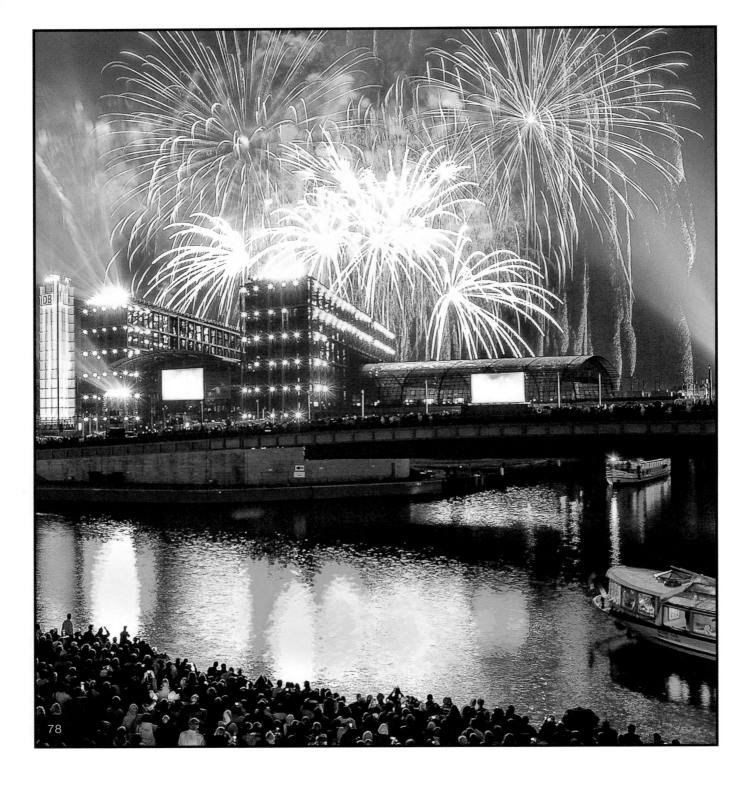

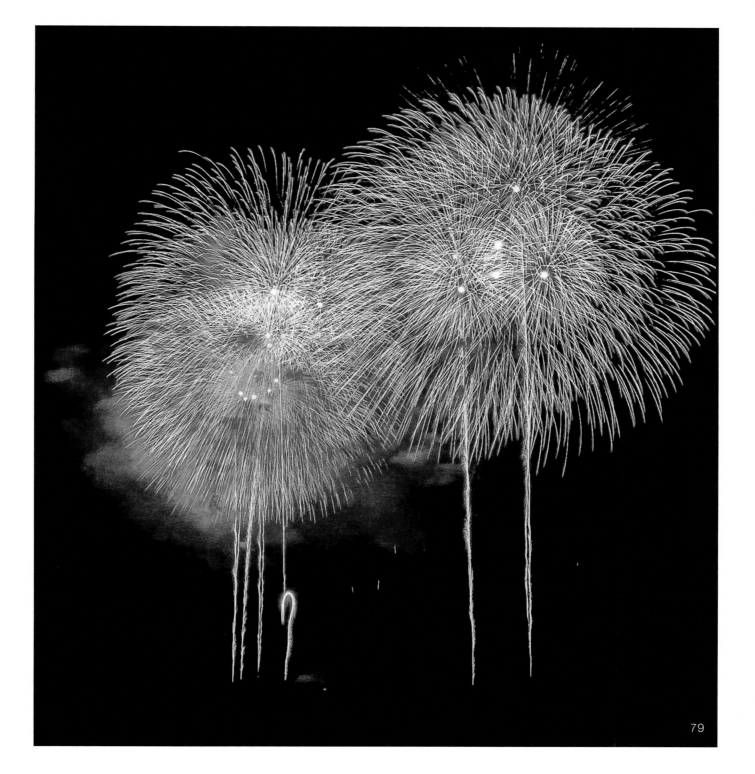

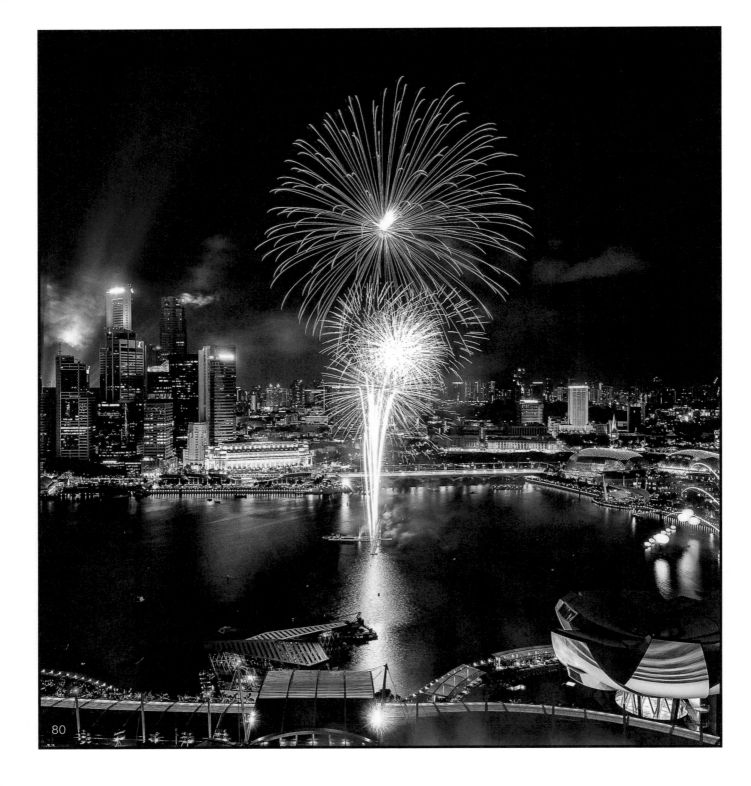

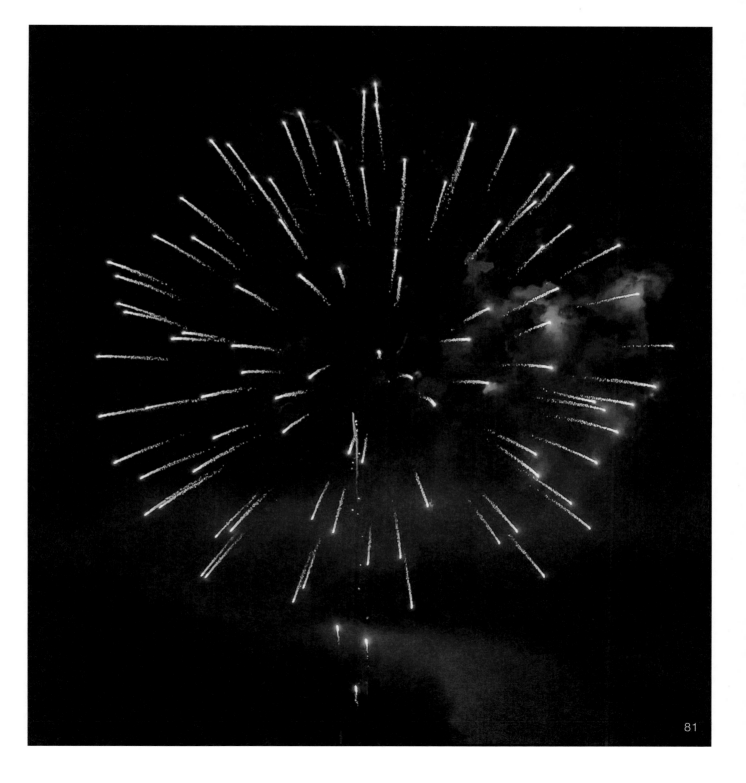

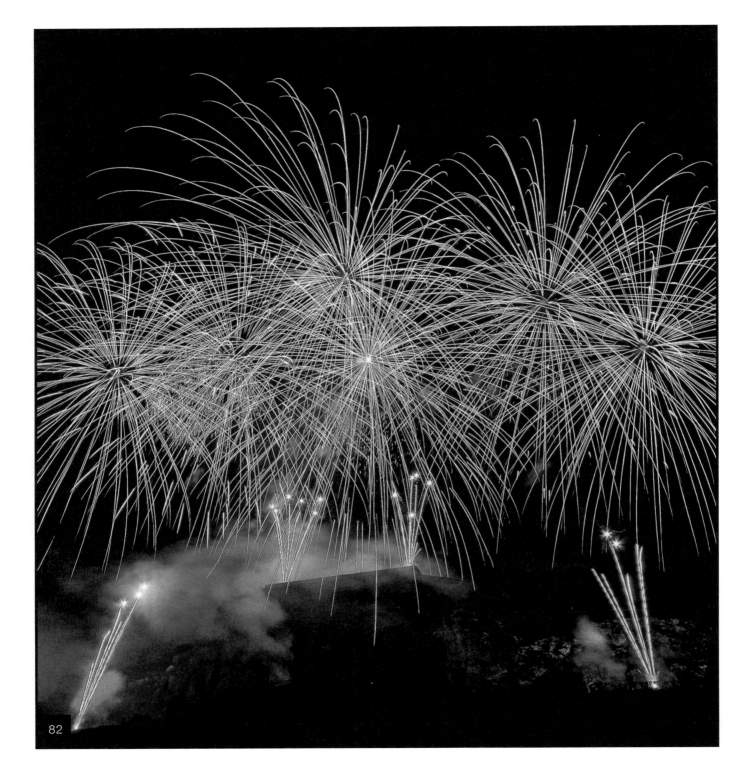

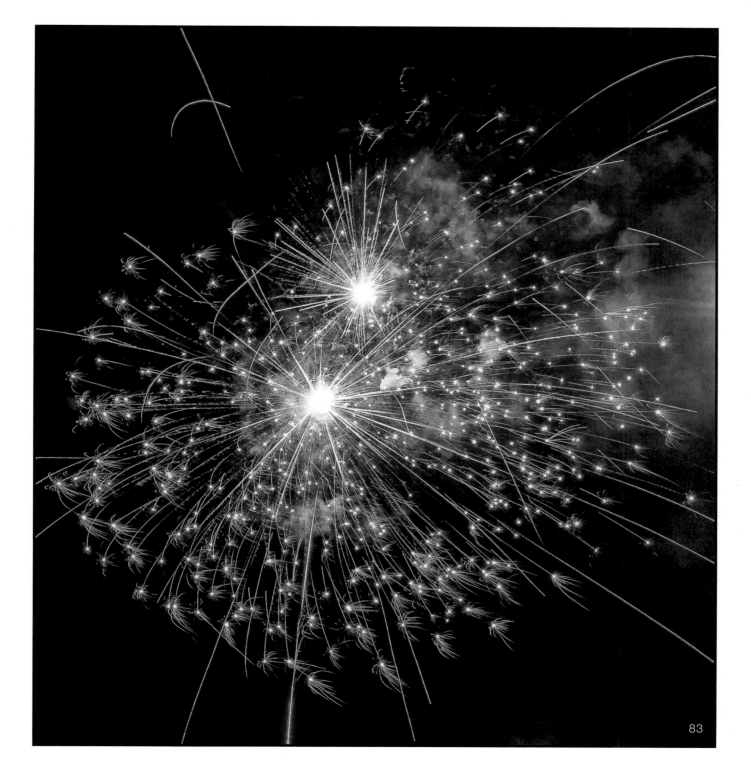

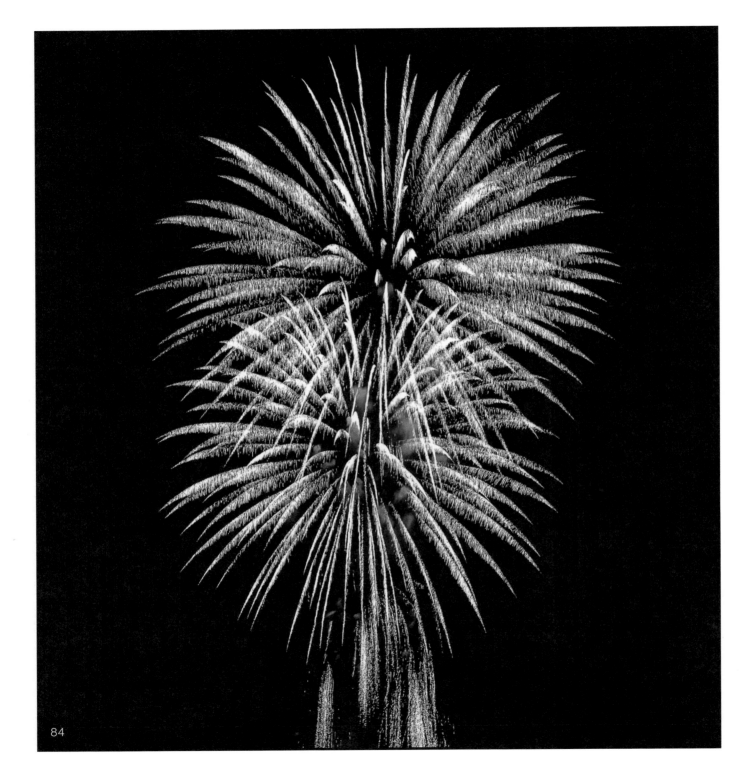

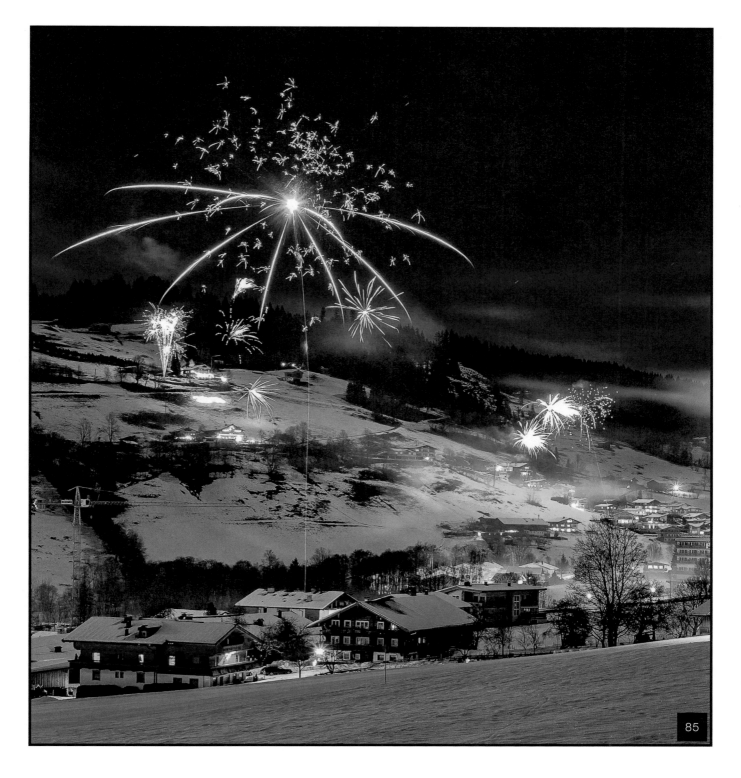

85

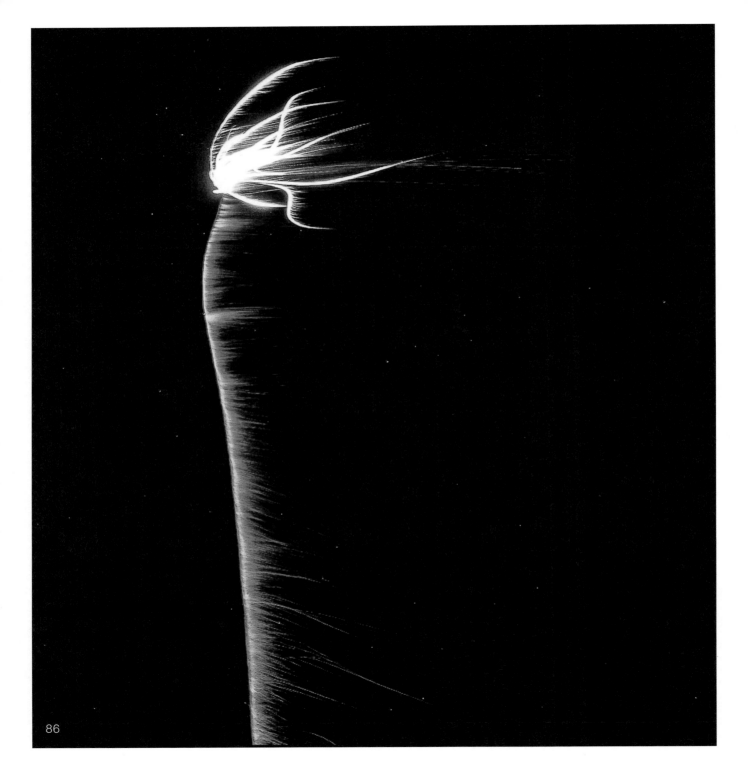

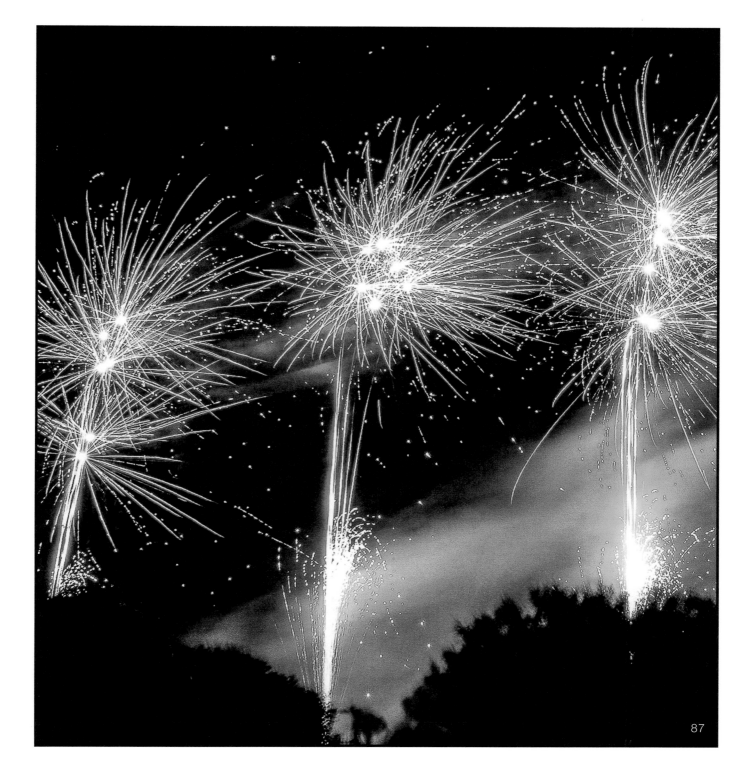

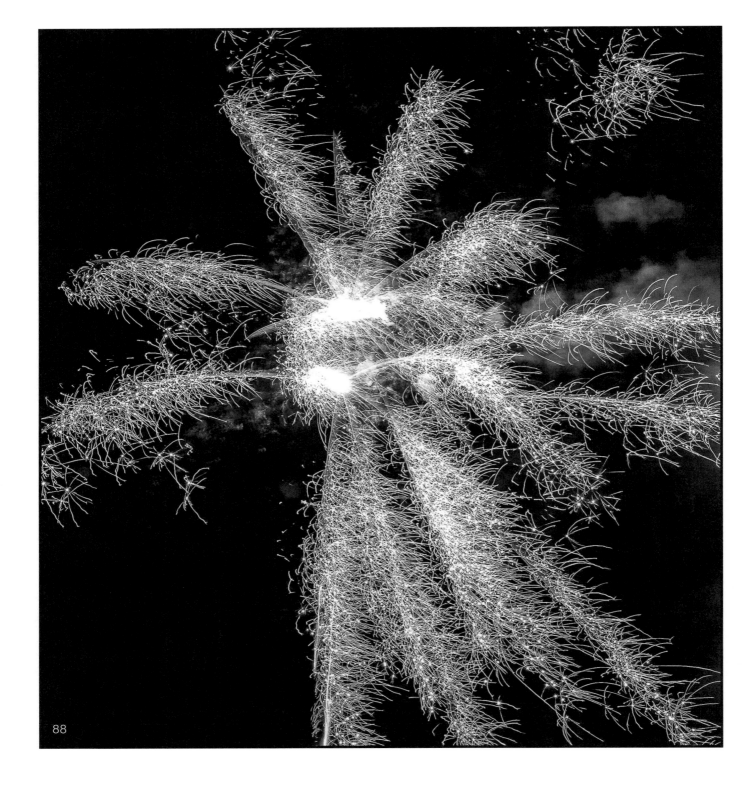

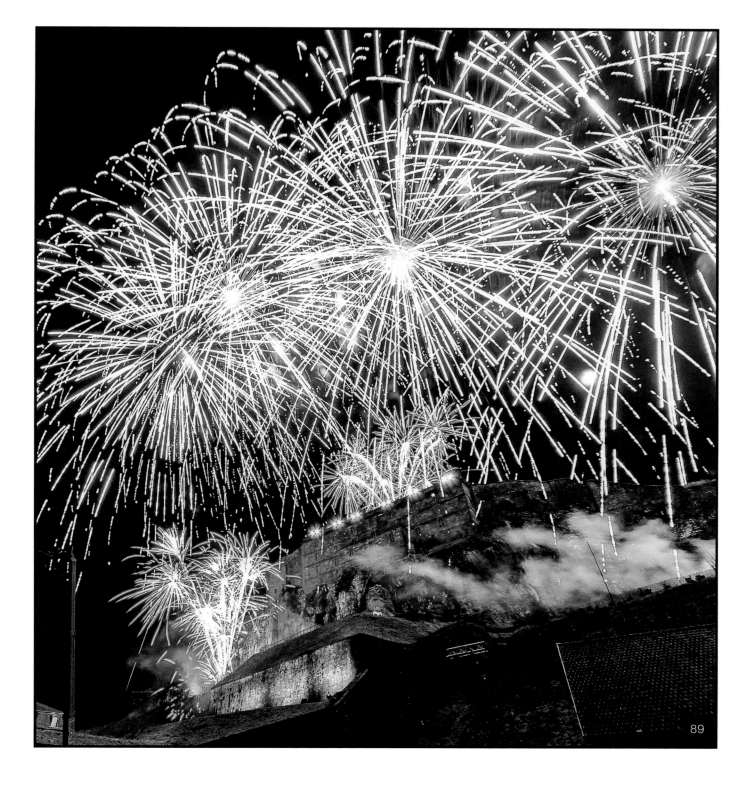

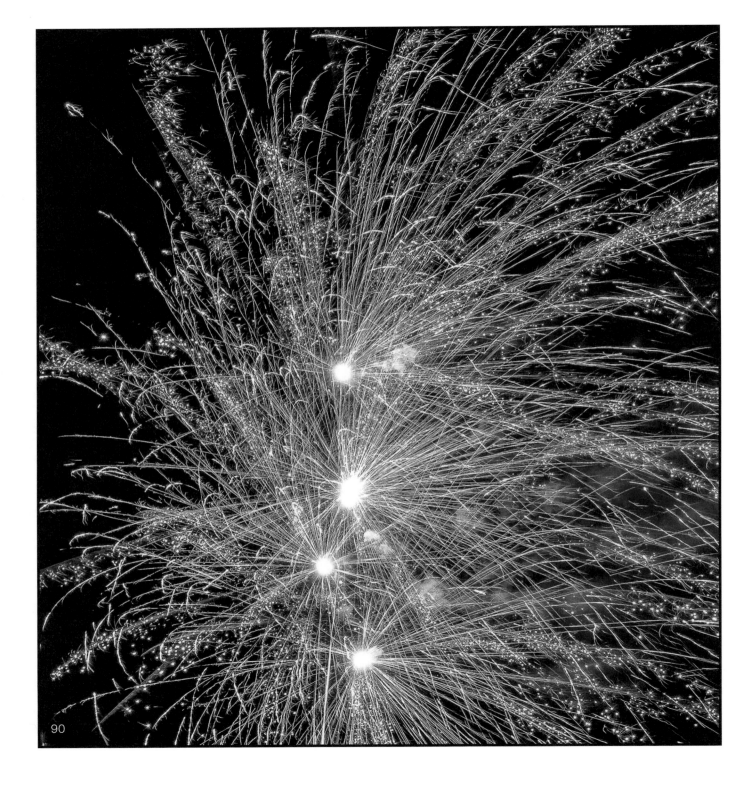

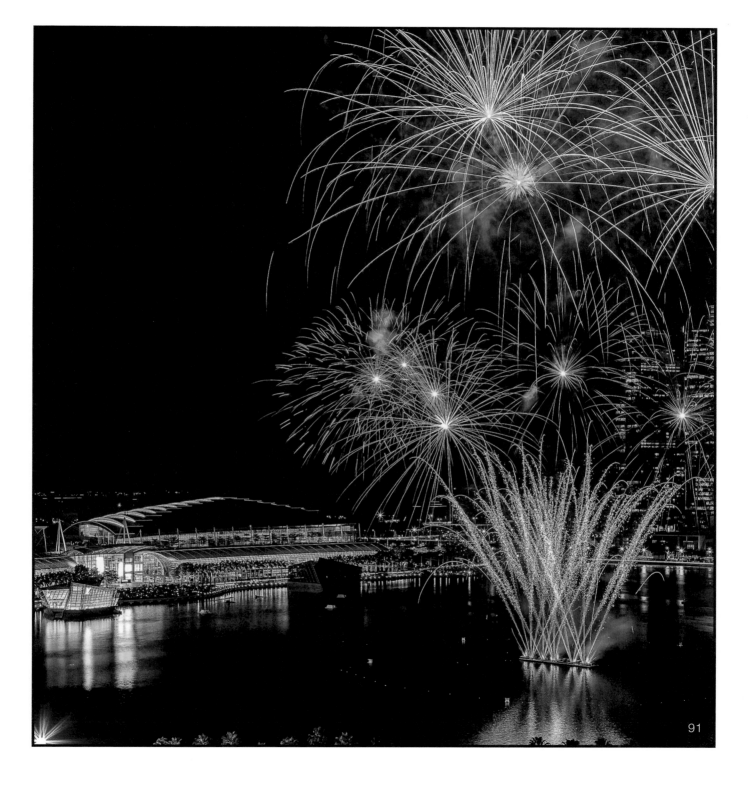

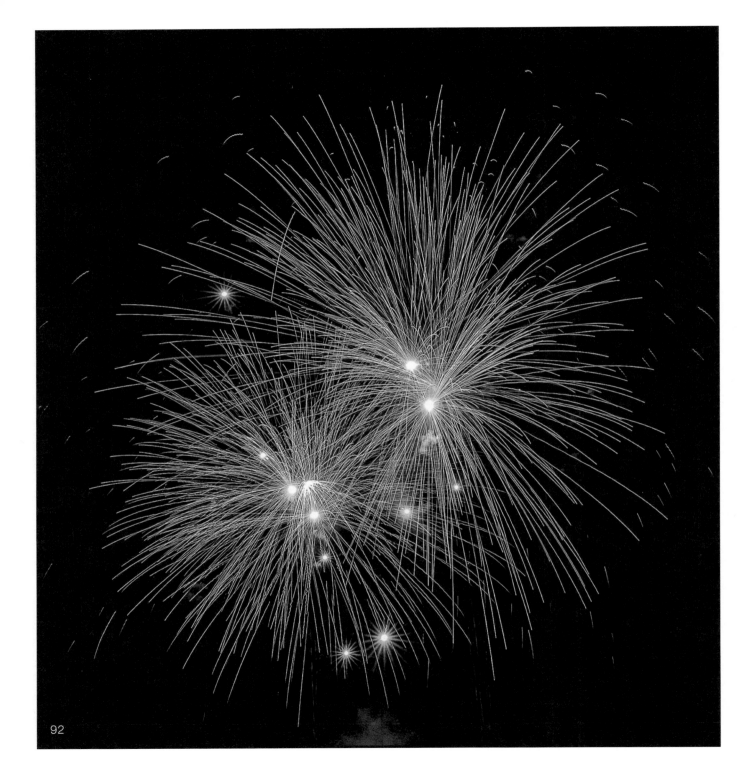

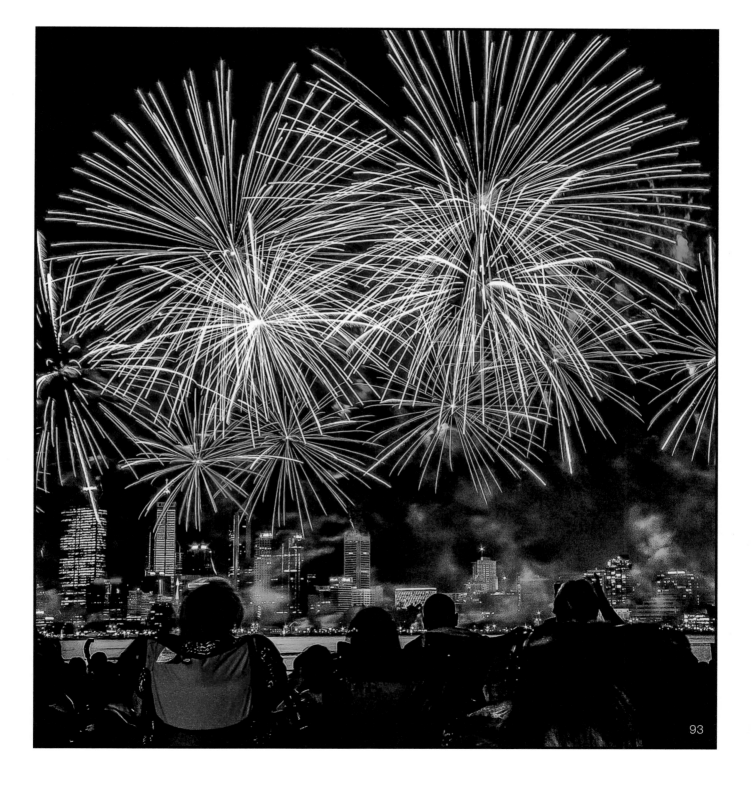

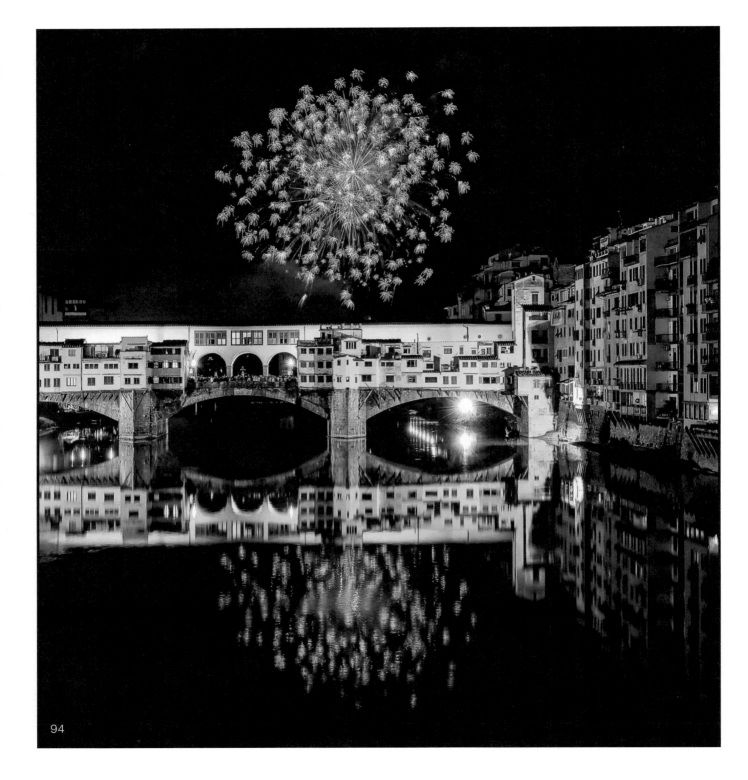

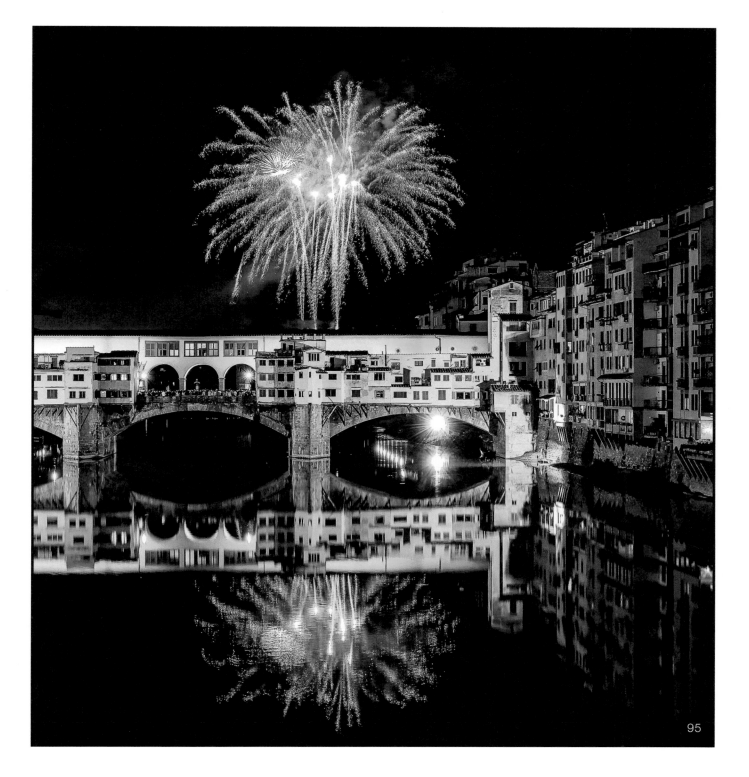

APPENDIX

Title: Firework two rockets
Date: 2013-01-01 01:23:53
Description: A picture of two exploding firework rockets.
Artist: Paul-Vincent Roll
Credit: Own work
Source: *https://commons.wikimedia.org/wiki/File:Firework_two_rockets.jpg*
License: Creative Commons Attribution-Share Alike 3.0 *https://creativecommons.org/licenses/by-sa/3.0*

Page: 11
Title: Feu d'artifice - 287
Date: 2015-07-14 21:24:38
Description: Fireworks in Annecy, France.
Artist: Medium69 (William Crochot)
Credit: Own work
Source: *https://commons.wikimedia.org/wiki/File:Feu_d'artifice_-_287.jpg*
License: Creative Commons Attribution-Share Alike 4.0 *https://creativecommons.org/licenses/by-sa/4.0*

Page: 12
Title: Feu d'artifice - 286
Date: 2015-07-14 21:24:03
Description: Fireworks in Annecy, France.
Artist: Medium69 (William Crochot)
Credit: Own work
Source: *https://commons.wikimedia.org/wiki/File:Feu_d'artifice_-_286.jpg*
License: Creative Commons Attribution-Share Alike 4.0 *https://creativecommons.org/licenses/by-sa/4.0*

Page: 13
Title: Feu d'artifice - 296
Date: 2015-07-14 21:26:54
Description: Fireworks in Annecy, France.
Artist: Medium69 (William Crochot)
Credit: Own work
Source: *https://commons.wikimedia.org/wiki/File:Feu_d'artifice_-_296.jpg*
License: Creative Commons Attribution-Share Alike 4.0 *https://creativecommons.org/licenses/by-sa/4.0*

Page: 14
Title: Feu d'artifice - 328
Date: 2015-07-14 21:37:54
Description: Fireworks in Annecy, France.
Artist: Medium69 (William Crochot)
Credit: Own work
Source: *https://commons.wikimedia.org/wiki/File:Feu_d'artifice_-_328.jpg*
License: Creative Commons Attribution-Share Alike 4.0 *https://creativecommons.org/licenses/by-sa/4.0*

Page: 15
Title: Ignis Brunensis Macedos Pirotecnia 2007
Date: 2007-05-30
Description: Contest performance on Brno dam of group Macedo´s Pirotecnia from Portugal
Artist: For use outside of Wikimedia projects, you have to credit also with hyperlink. For other licenses or terms of use contact me.
Credit: Own work
Source: *https://commons.wikimedia.org/wiki/File:Ignis_Brunensis_Macedos_Pirotecnia_2007.jpg*
License: Creative Commons Attribution-Share Alike 3.0 *https://creativecommons.org/licenses/by-sa/3.0*

Page: 16

Title: Pitten - Firework (01)
Date: 2010-12-05
Description: Firework
Artist: Steindy (talk) 00:21, 24 December 2014 (UTC)
Credit: Own work
Source: *https://commons.wikimedia.org/wiki/File:Pitten_-_Firework_(01).jpg*
License: Creative Commons Attribution-Share Alike 3.0 *https://creativecommons.org/licenses/by-sa/3.0*

Page: 17
Title: Fireworks5 amk
Date: 2007-08
Description: Fireworks
Artist: user:AngMoKio
Credit: Own work
Source: *https://commons.wikimedia.org/wiki/File:Fireworks5_amk.jpg*
License: Creative Commons Attribution-Share Alike 2.5 *https://creativecommons.org/licenses/by-sa/2.5*

Page: 18
Title: Feuerwerk Dreiländerbrücke
Date: 2007-06-30
Description: Fireworks for opening the Three Countries Bridge
Artist: Wladyslaw
Credit: Own work
Source: *https://commons.wikimedia.org/wiki/File:Feuerwerk_Dreiländerbrücke.jpg*
License: Creative Commons Attribution-Share Alike 3.0 *http://creativecommons.org/licenses/by-sa/3.0/*

Page: 19
Title: Feu d'artifice - 326
Date: 2015-07-14 21:37:31
Description: Fireworks

in Annecy, France.
Artist: Medium69 (William Crochot)
Credit: Own work
Source: _https://commons.wikimedia._
_org/wiki/File:Feu_d'artifice_-_326.jpg_
License: Creative Commons
Attribution-Share Alike 4.0
https://creativecommons.o
rg/licenses/by-sa/4.0

Page: 20
Title: Summerfest 2008
fireworks 7096
Date: 2008-06-26
Description: Fireworks on
the first day of Summerfest,
Milwaukee, Wisconsin
Artist: Dori
Credit: Own work
Source: _https://commons.wiki_
media.org/wiki/File:Summerfes
_t_2008_fireworks_7096.jpg_
License: Creative Commons
Attribution-Share Alike 3.0 us
https://creativecommons.org/lic
enses/by-sa/3.0/us/deed.en

Page: 21
Title: Feu d'artifice - 335
Date: 2015-07-14 21:41:16
Description: Fireworks
in Annecy, France.
Artist: Medium69 (William Crochot)
Credit: Own work
Source: _https://commons.wikimedia._
_org/wiki/File:Feu_d'artifice_-_335.jpg_
License: Creative Commons
Attribution-Share Alike 4.0
https://creativecommons.o
rg/licenses/by-sa/4.0

Page: 22
Title: Feu d'artifice - 301
Date: 2015-07-14 21:28:04
Description: Fireworks

in Annecy, France.
Artist: Medium69 (William Crochot)
Credit: Own work
Source: _https://commons.wikimedia._
_org/wiki/File:Feu_d'artifice_-_301.jpg_
License: Creative Commons
Attribution-Share Alike 4.0
https://creativecommons.o
rg/licenses/by-sa/4.0

Page: 23
Title: Marina-Bay Singapore
Firework-launching-CNY-2015-05
Date: 2015-02-18
Description: Marina Bay,
Singapore: Firework display at
midnight in Marina Bay, launching
the Chinese New Year 2015
Artist: CEphoto, Uwe Aranas
Credit: Own work
Source: _https://commons.wikimedia._
_org/wiki/File:Marina-Bay_Singapore_
Firework-launching-CNY-2015-05.jpg
License: Creative Commons
Attribution-Share Alike 3.0
https://creativecommons.o
rg/licenses/by-sa/3.0

Page: 24
Title: Marina-Bay Singapore
Firework-launching-CNY-2015-07
Date: 2015-02-18
Description: Marina Bay,
Singapore: Firework display at
midnight in Marina Bay, launching
the Chinese New Year 2015
Artist: CEphoto, Uwe Aranas
Credit: Own work
Source: _https://commons.wikimedia._
_org/wiki/File:Marina-Bay_Singapore_
Firework-launching-CNY-2015-07.jpg
License: Creative Commons
Attribution-Share Alike 3.0
https://creativecommons.o
rg/licenses/by-sa/3.0

Page: 25
Title: Wildschönau feiert
Neues Jahr 02
Date: 2013-01-01 00:05:22
Description: Firework at the New
Year's Eve in Niederau, Tyrol, Austria.
Artist: Ximeg
Credit: Own work
Source: _https://commons.wiki_
media.org/wiki/File:Wildschöna
_u_feiert_Neues_Jahr_02.jpg_
License: Creative Commons
Attribution-Share Alike 3.0
https://creativecommons.o
rg/licenses/by-sa/3.0

Page: 26
Title: Feu d'artifice - 336
Date: 2015-07-14 21:41:21
Description: Fireworks
in Annecy, France.
Artist: Medium69 (William Crochot)
Credit: Own work
Source: _https://commons.wikimedia._
_org/wiki/File:Feu_d'artifice_-_336.jpg_
License: Creative Commons
Attribution-Share Alike 4.0
https://creativecommons.o
rg/licenses/by-sa/4.0

Page: 27
Title: Fourth of July Fireworks
at Washington DC - 1
Date: 2011-07-04
Description: Fourth of July fireworks
seen across the Potomac River
at Washington, D.C., USA.
Artist: Joe Ravi
Credit: Own work
Source: _https://commons.wikimed_
_ia.org/wiki/File:Fourth_of_July_Fire_
_works_at_Washington_DC_-_1.jpg_
License: Creative Commons
Attribution-Share Alike 3.0
https://creativecommons.o

APPENDIX

Page: 55
Title: Feu d'artifice - 200
Date: 2015-07-13 21:54:32
Description: Fireworks in Annecy-le-Vieux, France.
Artist: Medium69 (William Crochot)
Credit: Own work
Source: https://commons.wikimedia.org/wiki/File:Feu_d'artifice_-_200.jpg
License: Creative Commons Attribution-Share Alike 4.0
https://creativecommons.org/licenses/by-sa/4.0

Page: 56
Title: Feu d'artifice - 201
Date: 2015-07-13 21:56:49
Description: Fireworks in Annecy-le-Vieux, France.
Artist: Medium69 (William Crochot)
Credit: Own work
Source: https://commons.wikimedia.org/wiki/File:Feu_d'artifice_-_201.jpg
License: Creative Commons Attribution-Share Alike 4.0
https://creativecommons.org/licenses/by-sa/4.0

Page: 57
Title: 200508 Firework of Lake of Annecy festival (363)
Source: https://commons.wikimedia.org/wiki/File:200508_Firework_of_Lake_of_Annecy_festival_(363).jpg
License: Creative Commons Attribution-Share Alike 3.0
http://creativecommons.org/licenses/by-sa/3.0/

Page: 58
Title: Feu d'artifice - 302
Date: 2015-07-14 21:28:12

Description: Fireworks in Annecy, France.
Artist: Medium69 (William Crochot)
Credit: Own work
Source: https://commons.wikimedia.org/wiki/File:Feu_d'artifice_-_302.jpg
License: Creative Commons Attribution-Share Alike 4.0
https://creativecommons.org/licenses/by-sa/4.0

Page: 59
Title: Feu d'artifice - 279
Date: 2015-07-14 21:21:53
Description: Fireworks in Annecy, France.
Artist: Medium69 (William Crochot)
Credit: Own work
Source: https://commons.wikimedia.org/wiki/File:Feu_d'artifice_-_279.jpg
License: Creative Commons Attribution-Share Alike 4.0
https://creativecommons.org/licenses/by-sa/4.0

Page: 60
Title: Wildschönau feiert Neues Jahr 03
Date: 2013-01-01 00:05:22
Description: Firework at the New Year's Eve in Niederau, Tyrol, Austria.
Artist: Ximeg
Credit: Own work
Source: https://commons.wikimedia.org/wiki/File:Wildschönau_feiert_Neues_Jahr_03.jpg
License: Creative Commons Attribution-Share Alike 3.0
https://creativecommons.org/licenses/by-sa/3.0

Page: 61
Title: Feu d'artifice - 308
Date: 2015-07-14 21:29:51
Description: Fireworks

in Annecy, France.
Artist: Medium69 (William Crochot)
Credit: Own work
Source: https://commons.wikimedia.org/wiki/File:Feu_d'artifice_-_308.jpg
License: Creative Commons Attribution-Share Alike 4.0
https://creativecommons.org/licenses/by-sa/4.0

Page: 62
Title: ദീപാവലി ആഘോഷം
Date: 2008-10-31
Description: ദീപാവലി ആഘോഷം
Artist: Santhoshj at Malayalam Wikipedia
Credit: Sreejithk2000
Source: https://commons.wikimedia.org/wiki/File:ദീപാവലി_ആഘോഷം.JPG
License: Creative Commons Attribution-Share Alike 3.0
https://creativecommons.org/licenses/by-sa/3.0

Page: 63
Title: Fireworks lugano 2011-2
Date: 2011-08-01 22:55:34
Description: Fireworks, Swiss National Day Aug 1st, 2011, Lugano, Switzerland.
Artist: Philippe Moret
Credit: Own work
Source: https://commons.wikimedia.org/wiki/File:Fireworks_lugano_2011-2.jpg
License: Creative Commons Attribution-Share Alike 4.0
https://creativecommons.org/licenses/by-sa/4.0

Page: 64
Title: 2014-01-01 00-11-24 feux-artifices-belfort
Date: 2014-01-01 00:11:24

Description: Feu d'artifice, à Belfort.
Artist: Thomas Bresson
Credit: Own work
Source: *https://commons.wikim edia.org/wiki/File:2014-01-01_00 -11-24_feux-artifices-belfort.jpg*
License: Creative Commons Attribution 3.0 *https://creativecommons .org/licenses/by/3.0*

Page: 65
Title: Feu d'artifice - 312
Date: 2015-07-14 21:33:01
Description: Fireworks in Annecy, France.
Artist: Medium69 (William Crochot)
Credit: Own work
Source: *https://commons.wikimedia. org/wiki/File:Feu_d'artifice_-_312.jpg*
License: Creative Commons Attribution-Share Alike 4.0 *https://creativecommons.o rg/licenses/by-sa/4.0*

Page: 66 *(cover image)*
Title: July 4th fireworks, Washington, D.C. (LOC)
Date: 2008-07-04
Description: July 4th fireworks, Washington, D.C. 2008 July 4. 1 photograph : digital, TIFF file, color. Washington, D.C., is a spectacular place to celebrate July 4th! The National Mall, with Washington D.C.'s monuments and the U.S. Capitol in the background, forms a beautiful and patriotic backdrop to America's Independence Day celebrations.Credit line: Carol M. Highsmith's America, Library of Congress, Prints and Photographs Division.Rights Info: No known restrictions on publication.Repository: Library of Congress, Prints and

Photographs Division, Washington, D.C. 20540 USA, hdl.loc.gov/loc.pnp/ pp.printMore information about the Highsmith Collection is available at hdl.loc.gov/loc.pnp/pp.highsm Call Number: LC-DIG-highsm- 04694
Artist: Carol M. Highsmith
Credit: This image is available from the United States Library of Congress's Prints and Photographs division under the digital ID highsm.04694.This tag does not indicate the copyright status of the attached work. A normal copyright tag is still required. See Commons:Licensing for more information.
Source: *https://commons.wikime dia.org/wiki/File:July_4th_firework s,_Washington,_D.C._(LOC).jpg*
License: Public domain

Page: 67
Title: Australia Day 2013 Perth 33
Date: 2013-01-26 14:23:09
Description: Australia Day Celebrations in Perth, WA - 26 January 2013
Artist: Kaoz69
Credit: Own work
Source: *https://commons.wi kimedia.org/wiki/File:Australi a_Day_2013_Perth_33.jpg*
License: Creative Commons Attribution-Share Alike 3.0 *https://creativecommons.o rg/licenses/by-sa/3.0*

Page: 68
Title: Feu d'artifice - 310
Date: 2015-07-14 21:32:13
Description: Fireworks in Annecy, France.
Artist: Medium69 (William Crochot)
Credit: Own work

Source: *https://commons.wikimedia. org/wiki/File:Feu_d'artifice_-_310.jpg*
License: Creative Commons Attribution-Share Alike 4.0 *https://creativecommons.o rg/licenses/by-sa/4.0*

Page: 69
Title: Feu d'artifice - 202
Date: 2015-07-13 21:58:15
Description: Fireworks in Annecy-le-Vieux, France.
Artist: Medium69 (William Crochot)
Credit: Own work
Source: *https://commons.wikimedia. org/wiki/File:Feu_d'artifice_-_202.jpg*
License: Creative Commons Attribution-Share Alike 4.0 *https://creativecommons.o rg/licenses/by-sa/4.0*

Page: 70
Title: Fireworks over Ponte Vecchio 2
Date: 2013-06-24 22:03:05
Description: Fireworks over Ponte Vecchio, Florence, Italy, part of UNESCO World Heritage Site Ref. Number 174
Artist: Martin Falbisoner
Credit: Own work
Source: *https://commons.wiki media.org/wiki/File:Fireworks_ over_Ponte_Vecchio_2.JPG*
License: Creative Commons Attribution-Share Alike 3.0 *https://creativecommons.o rg/licenses/by-sa/3.0*

Page: 71
Title: Wildschönau feiert Neues Jahr 06
Date: 2013-01-01 00:10:24
Description: Firework at the New Year's Eve in Niederau, Tyrol, Austria.
Artist: Ximeg

Credit: Own work
Source: _https://commons.wiki_
media.org/wiki/File:Wildschöna
_u_feiert_Neues_Jahr_06.jpg_
License: Creative Commons
Attribution-Share Alike 3.0
https://creativecommons.o
rg/licenses/by-sa/3.0

Page: 72
Title: Feu d'artifice - 331
Date: 2015-07-14 21:39:13
Description: Fireworks
in Annecy, France.
Artist: Medium69 (William Crochot)
Credit: Own work
Source: _https://commons.wikimedia._
_org/wiki/File:Feu_d'artifice_-_331.jpg_
License: Creative Commons
Attribution-Share Alike 4.0
https://creativecommons.o
rg/licenses/by-sa/4.0

Page: 73
Title: Feu d'artifice - 282
Date: 2015-07-14 21:22:29
Description: Fireworks
in Annecy, France.
Artist: Medium69 (William Crochot)
Credit: Own work
Source: _https://commons.wikimedia._
_org/wiki/File:Feu_d'artifice_-_282.jpg_
License: Creative Commons
Attribution-Share Alike 4.0
https://creativecommons.o
rg/licenses/by-sa/4.0

Page: 74
Title: Fourth of July Fireworks
at Washington DC - 2
Date: 2011-07-04
Description: Fourth of July fireworks
seen across the Potomac River
at Washington, D.C., USA.
Artist: Joe Ravi

Credit: Own work
Source: _https://commons.wikimed_
_ia.org/wiki/File:Fourth_of_July_Fire_
_works_at_Washington_DC_-_2.jpg_
License: Creative Commons
Attribution-Share Alike 3.0
https://creativecommons.o
rg/licenses/by-sa/3.0

Page: 75
Title: Feu d'artifice - 332
Date: 2015-07-14 21:40:38
Description: Fireworks
in Annecy, France.
Artist: Medium69 (William Crochot)
Credit: Own work
Source: _https://commons.wikimedia._
_org/wiki/File:Feu_d'artifice_-_332.jpg_
License: Creative Commons
Attribution-Share Alike 4.0
https://creativecommons.o
rg/licenses/by-sa/4.0

Page: 76
Title: Reflections of Earth 9
Date: 2008-01-11
Description: The IllumiNations:
Reflections of Earth fireworks show
at Epcot at Walt Disney World.
Artist: Benjamin D. Esham (bdesham)
Credit: This is a retouched picture,
which means that it has been
digitally altered from its original
version. Modifications: Denoising.
Modifications made by Bdesham.
Source: _https://commons.wikimedia.o_
_rg/wiki/File:Reflections_of_Earth_9.jpg_
License: Creative Commons
Attribution-Share Alike 3.0 us
https://creativecommons.org/lic
enses/by-sa/3.0/us/deed.en

Page: 77
Title: Feu d'artifice - 291
Date: 2015-07-14 21:25:33

Description: Fireworks
in Annecy, France.
Artist: Medium69 (William Crochot)
Credit: Own work
Source: _https://commons.wikimedia._
_org/wiki/File:Feu_d'artifice_-_291.jpg_
License: Creative Commons
Attribution-Share Alike 4.0
https://creativecommons.o
rg/licenses/by-sa/4.0

Page: 78
Title: Berlin Central Station
opening (2006)
Date: 2006-05-26
Description: Opening party for
Berlin Central Station. There
were about 500,000 visitors.
Artist: Jochen Teufel
Credit: Own work
Source: _https://commons.wikim_
_edia.org/wiki/File:Berlin_Centra_
_l_Station_opening_(2006).jpg_
License: Creative Commons
Attribution-Share Alike 3.0
https://creativecommons.o
rg/licenses/by-sa/3.0

Page: 79
Title: 2007 Nagaoka Festival 004
Date: 2007-08
Description: Fireworks
of Nagaoka Festival
Artist: Kropsoq
Credit: photo taken by Kropsoq
Source: _https://commons.wi_
_kimedia.org/wiki/File:2007_N_
_agaoka_Festival_004.jpg_
License: Creative Commons
Attribution-Share Alike 3.0
http://creativecommons.or
g/licenses/by-sa/3.0/

Page: 80
Title: 1 singapore national

Page: 89
Title: 2013-01-01 00-18-19-fireworks
Date: 2013-01-01 00:18:19
Description: This photograph was taken with a Nikon D300. Feu d'artifice à Belfort, à l'occasion du nouvel an.
Artist: Thomas Bresson
Credit: Own work
Source: https://commons.wikimedia.org/wiki/File:2013-01-01_00-18-19-fireworks.jpg
License: Creative Commons Attribution 3.0 https://creativecommons.org/licenses/by/3.0

Page: 90
Title: 2014 Fajerwerki w Kłodzku 05
Date: 2014-11-15 19:07:00
Description: Firerworks in Kłodzko
Artist: Jacek Halicki
Credit: Own work
Source: https://commons.wikimedia.org/wiki/File:2014_Fajerwerki_w_Kłodzku_05.jpg
License: Creative Commons Attribution-Share Alike 4.0 https://creativecommons.org/licenses/by-sa/4.0

Page: 91
Title: Marina-Bay Singapore Firework-launching-CNY-2015-06
Date: 2015-02-18
Description: Marina Bay, Singapore: Firework display at midnight in Marina Bay, launching the Chinese New Year 2015
Artist: CEphoto, Uwe Aranas
Credit: Own work
Source: https://commons.wikimedia.org/wiki/File:Marina-Bay_Singapore_Firework-launching-CNY-2015-06.jpg
License: Creative Commons Attribution-Share Alike 3.0 https://creativecommons.org/licenses/by-sa/3.0

Page: 92
Title: Feu d'artifice - 329
Date: 2015-07-14 21:38:36
Description: Fireworks in Annecy, France.
Artist: Medium69 (William Crochot)
Credit: Own work
Source: https://commons.wikimedia.org/wiki/File:Feu_d'artifice_-_329.jpg
License: Creative Commons Attribution-Share Alike 4.0 https://creativecommons.org/licenses/by-sa/4.0

Page: 93
Title: Australia Day 2013 Perth 28
Date: 2013-01-26 14:21:02
Description: Australia Day Celebrations in Perth, WA - 26 January 2013
Artist: Kaoz69
Credit: Own work
Source: https://commons.wikimedia.org/wiki/File:Australia_Day_2013_Perth_28.jpg
License: Creative Commons Attribution-Share Alike 3.0 https://creativecommons.org/licenses/by-sa/3.0

Page: 94
Title: Fireworks over Ponte Vecchio 3
Date: 2013-06-24 22:10:35
Description: Florence: Fireworks over Ponte Vecchio
Artist: Martin Falbisoner
Credit: Own work
Source: https://commons.wikimedia.org/wiki/File:Fireworks_over_Ponte_Vecchio_3.JPG
License: Creative Commons Attribution-Share Alike 3.0 https://creativecommons.org/licenses/by-sa/3.0

Page: 95
Title: Fireworks over Ponte Vecchio
Date: 2013-06-24 22:16:37
Description: Fireworks over Ponte Vecchio in Florence, Italy, part of UNESCO World Heritage Site Ref. Number 174
Artist: Martin Falbisoner
Credit: Own work
Source: https://commons.wikimedia.org/wiki/File:Fireworks_over_Ponte_Vecchio.JPG
License: Creative Commons Attribution-Share Alike 3.0 https://creativecommons.org/licenses/by-sa/3.0

Made in United States
Troutdale, OR
08/15/2023

12114436R00067